CRRN Study Guide:

Disclaimer: The information contained in this study guide is for general educational purposes only and is not intended as legal, medical, or professional advice. The authors and publishers have made every effort to ensure the accuracy and completeness of the information provided in this book. However, they cannot guarantee its accuracy or be held responsible for any errors, omissions, or inconsistencies.

Readers are advised to consult with a qualified professional, such as a legal or medical expert, before making any decisions or taking any actions based on the information contained in this study guide. The authors and publishers disclaim any liability or responsibility for any loss, damage, or injury that may arise from the use or misuse of the information provided in this book.

This study guide is not endorsed, sponsored, or affiliated with any organization, examination, or certification program mentioned herein. Any trademarks, logos, or service marks used in this book are the property of their respective owners and are used for identification purposes only.

By using this study guide, the reader acknowledges and agrees to the terms of this legal disclaimer and assumes full responsibility for their actions.

PAGE 2 Introduction.
PAGE 5 Rehabilitation Nursing Models and Theories.
PAGE 14 Functional Health Patterns in Rehabilitation Nursing.
PAGE 28 The Rehabilitation Nursing Process.
PAGE 37 Community Reintegration.
PAGE 48 Special Topics in Rehabilitation Nursing.
PAGE 62 - 167 Practice Exam Section.

INTRODUCTION:

Welcome to this comprehensive study guide designed to help you conquer the Certified Rehabilitation Registered Nurse (CRRN) Exam! We understand that pursuing a certification can be both an exciting and challenging journey. Our aim is to support your dreams, boost your confidence, and provide you with the essential tools and knowledge to achieve your professional goals.

In this study guide, we will walk you through the core concepts and principles of rehabilitation nursing, covering everything from models and theories to functional health patterns, the rehabilitation nursing process, and community reintegration. We have carefully crafted this guide to provide an in-depth understanding of the topics covered in the CRRN Exam, empowering you to excel and reach new heights in your nursing career.

As you delve into the content of this guide, you will find valuable information, practical examples, and real-world scenarios that will not only help you prepare for the exam but also enhance your skills in providing high-quality care to your patients.

We know that setbacks and fears may arise along the way, but we believe in your potential and dedication to succeed. This guide serves as a supportive companion that will help you overcome obstacles and turn your aspirations into reality. Together, we will help you build a solid foundation, strengthen your knowledge, and develop the confidence you need to excel in the CRRN Exam and beyond.

So, let's embark on this incredible journey together. We are here to provide you with the encouragement, guidance, and resources you need to turn your dreams into achievements. Remember, success is within your reach, and this study guide will be by your side every step of the way.

Let's dive into **an overview of the Certified Rehabilitation Registered Nurse (CRRN) Exam**, a crucial milestone in your journey toward becoming a certified expert in this field. We understand the significance of this exam in your career, and we're here to guide you every step of the way.

The CRRN Exam is designed to evaluate your knowledge and expertise in providing high-quality rehabilitation nursing care. Developed and administered by the Association of Rehabilitation Nurses (ARN), this certification exam is an excellent way to showcase your dedication and commitment to the profession, enhancing your credibility and opening new doors of opportunity.

The exam consists of 175 multiple-choice questions, which are divided into four main content domains:

1. Rehabilitation Nursing Models and Theories (6%)
2. Functional Health Patterns (58%)
3. The Rehabilitation Nursing Process (26%)
4. Community Reintegration (10%)

Each content domain covers a range of topics essential for rehabilitation nursing practice. From understanding the core concepts and principles to mastering the nursing process and facilitating community reintegration, the CRRN Exam aims to ensure you possess the skills and knowledge required to excel in this rewarding field.

The test duration is 3 hours, providing you with ample time to answer all questions. A passing score is determined using a criterion-referenced approach, which means your performance is measured against a predetermined standard rather than compared to other candidates.
To achieve success in the CRRN Exam, it's vital to develop a well-rounded understanding of the content domains and related topics. By studying this guide thoroughly and applying the principles and strategies covered, you will be well-prepared to tackle the exam and demonstrate your competence in rehabilitation nursing.

Remember, this is your chance to shine and prove your expertise in the field. Embrace the challenge, stay focused, and keep your eye on the prize. With determination, hard work, and the support of this study guide, you're on the path to achieving your CRRN certification and making a difference in the lives of your patients.

To help you get started on your journey towards becoming a Certified Rehabilitation Registered Nurse (CRRN), let's discuss the exam eligibility and application process.
Eligibility Criteria:
Before applying for the CRRN Exam, you must meet the following eligibility requirements set by the Association of Rehabilitation Nurses (ARN):
1. Current, unrestricted registered nurse (RN) license: You must hold an active and unrestricted RN license in the United States or its territories, or the legally recognized equivalent in another country.
2. Rehabilitation nursing experience: You need to have completed at least two years of practice as a registered nurse, with a minimum of 4,000 hours of rehabilitation nursing experience within the last five years. This experience should include direct patient care, education, administration, or research in rehabilitation nursing.

Application Process:
Once you have determined your eligibility, follow these steps to apply for the CRRN Exam:

1. Visit the ARN website: Access the ARN website (www.rehabnurse.org) to find detailed information about the CRRN Exam, including the application process, fees, and deadlines.
2. Complete the online application: Fill out the online application form, providing accurate and complete information about your professional background, nursing experience, and contact details.
3. Submit supporting documents: You may be required to submit documentation verifying your RN license and rehabilitation nursing experience, such as copies of your license, employment verification letters, or other relevant documents.
4. Pay the exam fee: Upon completing the application, you will need to pay the exam fee. Fees vary for ARN members and non-members, so be sure to check the latest fee structure on the ARN website.
5. Receive confirmation and schedule your exam: Once your application is reviewed and approved, you will receive an email confirmation with instructions on how to schedule your exam at a nearby testing center. The CRRN Exam is administered during specific testing windows throughout the year, so make sure to schedule your exam within the designated time frame.
6. Prepare for the exam: Use this study guide and other resources to prepare for the CRRN Exam, focusing on the content domains and relevant topics. Develop a study plan, practice with sample questions, and review key concepts to ensure your success on the exam day.

By following these steps and meeting the eligibility requirements, you will be well on your way to taking the CRRN Exam and advancing your career in rehabilitation nursing.

Rehabilitation Nursing Models and Theories:

Rehabilitation nursing models and theories play a crucial role in guiding rehabilitation nursing practice and enhancing patient outcomes. These models and theories provide a framework for understanding the complex needs of patients, guiding the nursing process, and fostering interdisciplinary collaboration. By integrating theoretical knowledge with clinical expertise, rehabilitation nurses can develop evidence-based care plans and interventions that promote optimal patient recovery and quality of life.

Models and theories in rehabilitation nursing help practitioners identify key factors that influence patients' abilities to function, adapt, and reintegrate into their communities. These factors may include physical, psychological, social, and environmental aspects of patients' lives. By understanding the interplay of these factors, rehabilitation nurses can design personalized care plans that address each patient's unique needs and preferences.

Furthermore, rehabilitation nursing models and theories emphasize the importance of patient-centered care, which involves actively engaging patients and their families in the decision-making process, setting realistic goals, and monitoring progress towards these goals. This patient-centered approach helps ensure that nursing interventions are tailored to each individual's needs, preferences, and values, ultimately leading to better patient satisfaction and improved outcomes.

In addition, models and theories in rehabilitation nursing provide a foundation for interdisciplinary collaboration, as they highlight the need for teamwork among various healthcare professionals, such as physicians, physical therapists, occupational therapists, and social workers. By working together within a common theoretical framework, these professionals can develop integrated care plans that address the multiple dimensions of patients' lives, leading to more effective and holistic care.

In summary, rehabilitation nursing models and theories are essential for guiding nursing practice and enhancing patient outcomes. They provide a framework for understanding the complex needs of patients, inform the nursing process, foster interdisciplinary collaboration, and promote patient-centered care. By incorporating these models and theories into their practice, rehabilitation nurses can help patients achieve their goals, optimize their functioning, and enhance their overall quality of life.

Key Principles of Rehabilitation Nursing
Rehabilitation nursing is a specialized field within nursing that focuses on helping patients with disabilities or chronic illnesses regain and maintain their highest level of functioning and independence. Several core principles underpin the practice of rehabilitation nursing, including patient-centered care, interdisciplinary collaboration, and goal-oriented interventions. These

principles guide rehabilitation nurses in providing comprehensive, individualized care to patients and their families.

1. Patient-centered care: Patient-centered care is at the heart of rehabilitation nursing. This principle emphasizes the importance of understanding and addressing each patient's unique needs, preferences, and values. Rehabilitation nurses actively engage patients and their families in the decision-making process, ensuring that care plans and interventions align with patients' goals and priorities. Patient-centered care fosters a strong therapeutic relationship, promotes patient autonomy, and ultimately leads to improved patient satisfaction and outcomes.
2. Interdisciplinary collaboration: Rehabilitation nursing recognizes the complex and multifaceted nature of patients' needs, which often require the expertise of various healthcare professionals. Interdisciplinary collaboration is a core principle of rehabilitation nursing that involves working closely with other healthcare providers, such as physicians, physical therapists, occupational therapists, speech therapists, and social workers. This collaborative approach ensures that care plans address all aspects of patients' lives and promote holistic care.
3. Goal-oriented interventions: Rehabilitation nursing focuses on helping patients achieve specific, measurable, and realistic goals that enhance their functioning and independence. Goal-oriented interventions are tailored to each patient's individual needs, taking into account their physical, psychological, social, and environmental circumstances. Rehabilitation nurses use evidence-based interventions to help patients reach their goals, regularly assess progress, and adjust care plans as needed to optimize patient outcomes.
4. Comprehensive assessment: A thorough and accurate assessment of each patient's needs and abilities is fundamental to rehabilitation nursing. Comprehensive assessment involves evaluating patients' physical, cognitive, emotional, and social functioning, as well as identifying potential barriers to recovery and reintegration. This information is used to develop personalized care plans that target patients' specific needs and goals.
5. Empowerment and education: Rehabilitation nursing aims to empower patients and their families by providing them with the knowledge, skills, and resources needed to manage their conditions effectively. This principle involves educating patients about their diagnoses, treatment options, and self-care strategies, as well as providing emotional support and encouragement throughout the rehabilitation process.

By adhering to these core principles, rehabilitation nurses can provide effective, compassionate care that helps patients regain their independence, improve their quality of life, and achieve their rehabilitation goals.

Overview of Nursing Theories Influencing Rehabilitation Nursing Practice

Nursing theories provide a foundation for understanding the complex dynamics of patient care and offer guidance for clinical practice. Several general nursing theories have influenced rehabilitation nursing, shaping its principles and interventions. Here, we will briefly introduce

Orem's Self-Care Deficit Theory, Roy's Adaptation Model, and Watson's Theory of Human Caring.

1. Orem's Self-Care Deficit Theory: Developed by Dorothea Orem, this theory asserts that individuals have a natural inclination and responsibility for self-care. However, when patients experience a self-care deficit due to illness or disability, nursing interventions are required to support them. Rehabilitation nursing adopts this principle, focusing on assisting patients in regaining or maintaining their self-care abilities and independence.
2. Roy's Adaptation Model: Sister Callista Roy's Adaptation Model emphasizes the importance of helping patients adapt to changes in their environment, health, or abilities. The model identifies four adaptive modes: physiological, self-concept, role function, and interdependence. Rehabilitation nursing incorporates these concepts by facilitating patients' adaptation to their new circumstances, supporting the development of new skills, and fostering resilience.
3. Watson's Theory of Human Caring: Jean Watson's theory highlights the significance of caring relationships between nurses and patients. According to this theory, nursing practice should be guided by values such as empathy, compassion, and respect for human dignity. Rehabilitation nursing embraces these values by fostering a caring environment, engaging patients in shared decision-making, and tailoring interventions to each patient's unique needs and preferences.

By incorporating the principles from these nursing theories, rehabilitation nursing practice can promote patient-centered care, empower individuals to regain or maintain their self-care abilities, and support patients' adaptation to changes in their health and abilities. Understanding these theories and their implications for rehabilitation nursing will help you provide holistic, compassionate, and effective care to your patients.

Theories Specific to Rehabilitation Nursing

Rehabilitation nursing is informed by several theories and models that are either unique to the field or particularly relevant for guiding practice. The Biopsychosocial Model, the Disablement Model, and the International Classification of Functioning, Disability, and Health (ICF) are three key frameworks that shape the understanding and approach of rehabilitation nurses in their work.

1. Biopsychosocial Model: The Biopsychosocial Model is a holistic approach that emphasizes the interplay of biological, psychological, and social factors in determining health and well-being. This model is highly relevant to rehabilitation nursing, as it recognizes that patients' recovery and reintegration into their communities depend on addressing not only their physical needs but also their psychological and social concerns. Rehabilitation nurses using this model assess patients' needs across all three domains and develop interventions that target each area to promote overall well-being and functioning.
2. Disablement Model: The Disablement Model focuses on the process through which health conditions or injuries result in disability, reduced functioning, and social participation restrictions. This model helps rehabilitation nurses understand the factors

contributing to patients' disabilities and guides them in developing interventions to minimize or prevent further limitations. The Disablement Model also emphasizes the importance of considering both personal and environmental factors in patients' lives, encouraging nurses to address barriers to successful rehabilitation and promote opportunities for reintegration.
   3. International Classification of Functioning, Disability, and Health (ICF): The ICF, developed by the World Health Organization (WHO), is a comprehensive classification system that provides a framework for understanding and measuring health and disability. The ICF considers three main components: body functions and structures, activities and participation, and environmental factors. Rehabilitation nurses use the ICF to assess patients' needs and abilities, set goals, and evaluate the effectiveness of interventions. By adopting the ICF, rehabilitation nursing practice becomes more standardized, allowing for improved communication and collaboration among healthcare professionals and better comparisons of patient outcomes across different settings.

These theories and models are essential for guiding rehabilitation nursing practice, as they provide a comprehensive and nuanced understanding of the factors that influence patients' recovery and reintegration. By incorporating these frameworks into their work, rehabilitation nurses can develop targeted, evidence-based interventions that address patients' unique needs and promote optimal functioning and quality of life.

Application of Theories in Rehabilitation Nursing Practice

Rehabilitation nursing theories and models play a crucial role in guiding clinical practice across various settings, including acute care, subacute care, outpatient clinics, and home care. In each of these environments, rehabilitation nurses apply these frameworks to assess patients, develop care plans, and implement interventions that address patients' unique needs and promote optimal functioning and quality of life.
   1. Acute care: In acute care settings, rehabilitation nurses focus on stabilizing patients' medical conditions and initiating the rehabilitation process as early as possible. They employ the Biopsychosocial Model, Disablement Model, and ICF to identify patients' immediate needs, develop goals, and provide interventions that promote recovery and prevent complications. This may include addressing patients' mobility issues, managing symptoms, and providing emotional support.
   2. Subacute care: Subacute care settings, such as skilled nursing facilities, serve patients who require a higher level of care than outpatient services but do not need the intensity of acute care. Rehabilitation nurses in these environments use the theories and models to develop comprehensive care plans that address patients' physical, cognitive, and emotional needs. Interventions may include pain management, mobility training, and caregiver education.
   3. Outpatient clinics: In outpatient settings, rehabilitation nurses collaborate with an interdisciplinary team to provide ongoing, coordinated care to patients who have transitioned from inpatient settings or are managing chronic conditions. They apply the

nursing theories and models to assess patients' progress, adjust care plans as needed, and deliver targeted interventions that support patients' continued recovery and independence. This can involve coordinating therapy services, providing patient education, and monitoring patients' overall health.
4. Home care: Rehabilitation nurses working in home care settings provide care to patients in their own homes, focusing on helping them adapt to their environment and maintain their independence. By applying the nursing theories and models, they assess patients' needs, develop individualized care plans, and implement interventions that promote safety, functioning, and quality of life. Home care interventions may include assistance with activities of daily living, medication management, and caregiver support.

By applying rehabilitation nursing theories and models across these diverse practice settings, nurses can ensure that patients receive consistent, evidence-based care that addresses their unique needs and promotes their recovery, functioning, and well-being.

Interdisciplinary Collaboration in Rehabilitation Nursing

Rehabilitation nursing models and theories play a vital role in promoting interdisciplinary teamwork and collaboration among healthcare professionals. As rehabilitation is a complex process requiring the expertise of various disciplines, effective communication and cooperation are essential for achieving optimal patient outcomes. Rehabilitation nursing models and theories, such as the Biopsychosocial Model, the Disablement Model, and the International Classification of Functioning, Disability, and Health (ICF), facilitate this interdisciplinary approach by providing a common language and framework for understanding patients' needs and goals.

1. Common language and understanding: Rehabilitation nursing models and theories offer a shared understanding of the factors that influence patients' health and functioning, allowing healthcare professionals from different disciplines to communicate effectively and work towards shared goals. For instance, the Biopsychosocial Model highlights the interplay of biological, psychological, and social factors, enabling team members to appreciate the importance of addressing each of these domains in patient care.
2. Comprehensive assessment and goal-setting: The use of comprehensive frameworks, such as the ICF, enables rehabilitation nurses and other healthcare professionals to conduct thorough assessments of patients' needs, abilities, and environmental factors. This facilitates the development of collaborative, patient-centered care plans that address each patient's unique circumstances and promote optimal functioning and quality of life.
3. Coordinated interventions: Rehabilitation nursing models and theories emphasize the importance of interdisciplinary collaboration in implementing interventions and monitoring patients' progress. By adopting these frameworks, rehabilitation nurses can work closely with physicians, physical therapists, occupational therapists, and social workers to deliver coordinated care that addresses patients' physical, cognitive, and emotional needs.
4. Evaluation and adaptation: As rehabilitation is an ongoing process, the use of nursing models and theories supports the continuous evaluation of patients' progress and the

adaptation of care plans as needed. This fosters a dynamic, collaborative approach among healthcare professionals, ensuring that patients receive the most appropriate and effective interventions throughout their rehabilitation journey.

In summary, rehabilitation nursing models and theories serve as the foundation for interdisciplinary collaboration in the field, fostering effective communication, comprehensive assessment, coordinated care, and ongoing evaluation among healthcare professionals. By embracing these frameworks, rehabilitation nurses and their colleagues can work together to provide holistic, patient-centered care that promotes optimal recovery, functioning, and well-being for individuals with disabilities or chronic health conditions.

The Role of Theories in Patient Assessment and Goal Setting

Rehabilitation nursing theories play a pivotal role in guiding the assessment process, goal setting, and the development of individualized care plans for patients with disabilities or chronic conditions. These theories, such as the Biopsychosocial Model, the Disablement Model, and the International Classification of Functioning, Disability, and Health (ICF), provide a comprehensive framework that informs the way rehabilitation nurses approach patient care.

1. Comprehensive patient assessment: Rehabilitation nursing theories emphasize the importance of conducting a thorough assessment that takes into account the patient's physical, psychological, and social needs. The Biopsychosocial Model, for instance, encourages nurses to explore the interplay of biological, psychological, and social factors influencing patients' health and well-being. This comprehensive assessment enables nurses to identify the specific needs and barriers that patients face in their recovery journey.
2. Goal setting: The Disablement Model and the ICF provide a structure for setting realistic, achievable goals based on patients' individual needs, abilities, and environmental factors. By using these frameworks, rehabilitation nurses can work with patients and their families to establish short-term and long-term goals that are patient-centered and focused on improving functioning, participation, and quality of life.
3. Individualized care plans: Rehabilitation nursing theories guide the development of tailored care plans that address the unique needs of each patient. These plans incorporate the findings from the comprehensive assessment and the established goals, outlining targeted interventions that target patients' specific challenges and promote their recovery and reintegration. The care plans also consider the interdisciplinary nature of rehabilitation, outlining the roles and responsibilities of each healthcare professional involved in the patient's care.
4. Ongoing evaluation and adaptation: The application of rehabilitation nursing theories supports the continuous monitoring of patients' progress and the adaptation of care plans as needed. By using these frameworks, nurses can evaluate the effectiveness of interventions, identify areas for improvement, and adjust goals and care plans to ensure that patients continue to receive the most appropriate and effective care throughout their rehabilitation journey.

In conclusion, rehabilitation nursing theories serve as the foundation for patient assessment, goal setting, and the development of individualized care plans. By embracing these frameworks, rehabilitation nurses can provide holistic, patient-centered care that addresses the unique needs of individuals with disabilities or chronic conditions, ultimately promoting their recovery, functioning, and well-being.

Theories and Evidence-Based Practice in Rehabilitation Nursing

The relationship between rehabilitation nursing theories and evidence-based practice is an essential aspect of providing high-quality care. These theories, such as the Biopsychosocial Model, the Disablement Model, and the International Classification of Functioning, Disability, and Health (ICF), provide a foundation for understanding the factors that influence patient outcomes. Evidence-based practice, on the other hand, involves integrating the best available research evidence with clinical expertise and patient preferences to guide nursing interventions. Together, they work synergistically to optimize patient care and promote recovery.

1. Informing nursing interventions: Rehabilitation nursing theories offer a framework that helps nurses understand the complex needs of patients with disabilities or chronic conditions. Evidence-based practice builds on this foundation by utilizing research findings to inform and refine nursing interventions. By integrating theoretical knowledge with empirical evidence, rehabilitation nurses can develop more effective, targeted interventions that address the specific challenges faced by their patients.
2. Enhancing patient outcomes: The combination of rehabilitation nursing theories and evidence-based practice enables nurses to make well-informed decisions about patient care. This ensures that interventions are grounded in both sound theoretical principles and empirical evidence, resulting in improved patient outcomes. Through the ongoing evaluation of evidence, nurses can continually refine their practice to better meet the needs of their patients and promote optimal recovery, functioning, and well-being.
3. Fostering professional development: Engaging in evidence-based practice encourages rehabilitation nurses to stay current with the latest research findings and advances in their field. This commitment to lifelong learning and professional growth enhances their clinical expertise and supports their ability to provide high-quality, patient-centered care.
4. Promoting interdisciplinary collaboration: The integration of rehabilitation nursing theories and evidence-based practice also supports interdisciplinary collaboration among healthcare professionals. By utilizing a common language and framework, nurses can effectively communicate with other team members and advocate for evidence-based interventions that align with the shared goals of the interdisciplinary team.

In summary, the relationship between rehabilitation nursing theories and evidence-based practice is critical for ensuring high-quality, effective care for patients with disabilities or chronic conditions. By incorporating theoretical frameworks with research evidence, rehabilitation nurses can develop targeted interventions, improve patient outcomes, foster professional development, and promote interdisciplinary collaboration within the healthcare team.

Ethical Considerations in Rehabilitation Nursing Practice

In the context of rehabilitation nursing, ethical principles and dilemmas often arise, given the unique challenges faced by patients with disabilities or chronic conditions. By understanding and applying nursing theories, rehabilitation nurses can better navigate these ethical considerations and make informed decisions that uphold the highest standards of patient care.

1. Ethical principles: The foundation of ethical nursing practice is built on several key principles, including autonomy, beneficence, nonmaleficence, justice, and fidelity. These principles serve as a guide for rehabilitation nurses as they strive to provide compassionate, patient-centered care while respecting the rights and dignity of their patients.
2. Autonomy and patient-centered care: One of the primary ethical considerations in rehabilitation nursing is respecting and promoting patient autonomy. Nursing theories, such as the Biopsychosocial Model, emphasize the importance of patient-centered care, which involves collaborating with patients to establish goals and develop care plans that align with their values and preferences.
3. Balancing beneficence and nonmaleficence: Rehabilitation nurses must carefully weigh the potential benefits and risks of various interventions to ensure they are acting in the best interests of their patients. Nursing theories can help guide this decision-making process by providing a comprehensive framework for understanding patients' needs and preferences, as well as the potential outcomes of different treatment options.
4. Justice and resource allocation: In rehabilitation nursing, ethical dilemmas may arise surrounding the fair distribution of resources and access to care. Nurses can draw on theories like the Disablement Model and the International Classification of Functioning, Disability, and Health (ICF) to advocate for equitable treatment and allocation of resources for their patients, ensuring that care is provided based on individual needs and potential for improvement.
5. Ethical decision-making: When faced with complex ethical dilemmas, rehabilitation nurses can turn to nursing theories as a source of guidance and support. These theories can help nurses to consider the various factors influencing their patients' well-being, as well as the potential consequences of different courses of action. By integrating theoretical knowledge with clinical expertise and patient preferences, nurses can make well-informed, ethical decisions that promote the best possible outcomes for their patients.

In conclusion, ethical considerations are an integral part of rehabilitation nursing practice. By applying nursing theories and adhering to ethical principles, rehabilitation nurses can navigate the challenges and dilemmas that may arise in their work, ultimately providing compassionate, patient-centered care that upholds the highest standards of ethical practice.

Throughout this chapter, we have explored the significance of rehabilitation nursing theories and models in guiding nursing practice, informing evidence-based interventions, fostering interdisciplinary collaboration, and addressing ethical considerations. In conclusion, the ongoing importance of these theories cannot be overstated, as they play a crucial role in shaping the future of the profession and enhancing patient outcomes.

Key points covered in this chapter include:
1. The importance of rehabilitation nursing models and theories in guiding practice and enhancing patient outcomes.
2. The foundational principles of rehabilitation nursing, such as patient-centered care, interdisciplinary collaboration, and goal-oriented interventions.
3. An overview of general nursing theories and their influence on rehabilitation nursing practice.
4. Theories and models specific to rehabilitation nursing and their applications in various practice settings.
5. The role of theories in patient assessment, goal setting, and individualized care planning.
6. The relationship between rehabilitation nursing theories and evidence-based practice.
7. Ethical considerations in rehabilitation nursing and the role of theories in ethical decision-making.

As we look towards the future of rehabilitation nursing, the continued refinement and application of these theories and models will be essential for advancing the profession and ensuring the highest quality of care for patients with disabilities and chronic conditions. This includess

1. Ongoing research and development of new theories: As the field of rehabilitation nursing continues to evolve, it is essential to develop and refine theories and models that address emerging challenges and opportunities in patient care.
2. Integration of technology and innovation: As new technologies and innovative approaches to care become more prevalent, rehabilitation nursing theories will need to adapt and incorporate these advances into their frameworks to guide nursing practice effectively.
3. Continued emphasis on interdisciplinary collaboration: Rehabilitation nursing theories will continue to play a critical role in fostering effective teamwork and collaboration among healthcare professionals, ensuring that patients receive comprehensive, coordinated care.
4. Addressing health disparities and promoting equity: Rehabilitation nursing theories and models can help to identify and address health disparities among different patient populations, promoting equitable access to care and improved outcomes for all patients.
5. Lifelong learning and professional development: Rehabilitation nurses must remain committed to ongoing education and professional growth, continually refining their understanding and application of nursing theories to provide the best possible care for their patients.

In summary, rehabilitation nursing theories and models are vital for guiding practice, promoting evidence-based care, fostering interdisciplinary collaboration, and addressing ethical considerations. As we look towards the future, these theories will continue to shape the profession, driving improvements in patient outcomes and advancing the field of rehabilitation nursing.

Functional Health Patterns in Rehabilitation Nursing:

Functional health patterns are a systematic approach to understanding and assessing various aspects of a patient's health, functioning, and well-being. In rehabilitation nursing, functional health patterns play a vital role in identifying patients' strengths, limitations, and areas for improvement, which ultimately helps develop individualized care plans to promote optimal recovery and rehabilitation outcomes.

The concept of functional health patterns was first introduced by Marjory Gordon, a nursing theorist, in 1987. The framework consists of 11 interrelated patterns that encompass a wide range of physical, psychological, and social factors affecting a patient's health. These patterns provide a comprehensive and holistic perspective on the patient's overall health status, enabling rehabilitation nurses to address their unique needs and challenges more effectively.

In the context of rehabilitation nursing, functional health patterns are particularly valuable because they:

1. Facilitate a comprehensive assessment: By considering all aspects of a patient's health, functional health patterns enable rehabilitation nurses to gain a deeper understanding of the patient's condition, needs, and potential barriers to recovery.
2. Guide individualized care planning: By identifying strengths and limitations in each functional health pattern, rehabilitation nurses can develop targeted interventions and strategies to enhance the patient's recovery and overall well-being.
3. Promote interdisciplinary collaboration: Functional health patterns encourage a team-based approach to care, as they involve the input of various healthcare professionals, such as physicians, physical therapists, occupational therapists, and social workers, to address the patient's diverse needs.
4. Support ongoing evaluation and monitoring: By using functional health patterns as a framework for assessment, rehabilitation nurses can track the patient's progress over time, allowing for adjustments to the care plan as needed.
5. Foster patient-centered care: Functional health patterns emphasize the importance of considering the patient's unique experiences, preferences, and goals in the rehabilitation process, which helps to ensure that care is tailored to their individual needs and priorities.

In summary, functional health patterns provide a valuable framework for assessing and addressing the diverse needs of patients in rehabilitation nursing. By considering all aspects of a patient's health and functioning, rehabilitation nurses can develop targeted and individualized care plans to support optimal recovery and enhance overall well-being.

Gordon's Functional Health Patterns: Relevance to Rehabilitation Nursing Practice

Marjory Gordon's Functional Health Patterns framework is an essential tool in rehabilitation nursing practice. Introduced in 1987, this framework comprises 11 interrelated patterns that provide a systematic and comprehensive approach to assessing various aspects of a patient's health, functioning, and well-being. These patterns encompass a wide range of physical, psychological, and social factors that influence a patient's health status.

The 11 functional health patterns are:
1. Health Perception-Health Management
2. Nutritional-Metabolic
3. Elimination
4. Activity-Exercise
5. Sleep-Rest
6. Cognitive-Perceptual
7. Self-Perception-Self-Concept
8. Role-Relationship
9. Sexuality-Reproductive
10. Coping-Stress Tolerance
11. Value-Belief

In rehabilitation nursing practice, Gordon's Functional Health Patterns framework is highly relevant for several reasons:

1. Comprehensive Assessment: The framework enables nurses to conduct a thorough and holistic evaluation of a patient's health status, considering all aspects of their well-being. This comprehensive assessment allows for the identification of specific needs, strengths, and limitations, which is crucial for developing individualized care plans.
2. Individualized Care Planning: By focusing on each functional health pattern, rehabilitation nurses can create targeted interventions and strategies that address the unique needs and challenges of each patient. This individualized approach ultimately leads to better recovery and rehabilitation outcomes.
3. Interdisciplinary Collaboration: The framework encourages a team-based approach to care, as it requires the input of various healthcare professionals to address the patient's diverse needs. This collaboration ensures that all aspects of the patient's health and well-being are considered and addressed effectively.
4. Ongoing Evaluation and Monitoring: Gordon's Functional Health Patterns provide a consistent framework for monitoring and evaluating a patient's progress over time. This consistency allows for adjustments to the care plan as needed and ensures that the patient's needs are continually met.
5. Patient-Centered Care: The framework emphasizes the importance of understanding and considering the patient's unique experiences, preferences, and goals in the rehabilitation process. This patient-centered approach ensures that care is tailored to each individual's needs and priorities.

In summary, Marjory Gordon's Functional Health Patterns framework is a valuable and relevant tool in rehabilitation nursing practice. By providing a comprehensive and systematic approach to assessing and addressing the diverse needs of patients, this framework enables nurses to develop individualized care plans that support optimal recovery and enhance overall well-being.

Health Perception-Health Management Pattern: Importance in Rehabilitation Nursing

The Health Perception-Health Management Pattern is the first of Marjory Gordon's Functional Health Patterns. This pattern focuses on a patient's understanding of their health status, their beliefs about illness and wellness, and their ability to manage their care effectively. In the context of rehabilitation nursing, assessing the Health Perception-Health Management Pattern is crucial for several reasons:

1. Identifying Health Beliefs: Understanding a patient's beliefs about their health status, illness, and recovery is essential in developing an effective care plan. Patients with a positive outlook and realistic expectations tend to engage more actively in their rehabilitation process, which can lead to better outcomes.
2. Recognizing Barriers to Care: Assessing this pattern allows rehabilitation nurses to identify potential barriers that might impede a patient's adherence to their care plan. These barriers can include lack of understanding, cultural beliefs, financial constraints, or inadequate support systems. By recognizing these challenges, nurses can develop interventions and strategies to address them and facilitate patient adherence to their care plan.
3. Assessing Self-Care Skills: Rehabilitation often involves teaching patients self-care skills, such as managing medications, performing exercises, or using assistive devices. Evaluating a patient's ability and willingness to engage in self-care activities is crucial to tailoring interventions and ensuring a successful rehabilitation process.
4. Monitoring Progress and Adjusting Care Plans: As patients progress through the rehabilitation process, their health perceptions and management abilities may change. Regular assessment of this pattern enables rehabilitation nurses to adjust care plans accordingly, ensuring that patients continue to receive the support they need.
5. Promoting Health and Wellness: A patient's health perception and management skills can impact their overall health and well-being beyond the immediate rehabilitation setting. By fostering positive health beliefs and effective self-care skills, rehabilitation nurses can promote long-term health and wellness for their patients.

In summary, the Health Perception-Health Management Pattern is an essential aspect of rehabilitation nursing assessment. By evaluating a patient's understanding of their health status and ability to manage their care, nurses can develop targeted interventions that support active participation in the rehabilitation process, address barriers to care, and promote long-term health and wellness.

Nutritional-Metabolic Pattern: Role in Rehabilitation Nursing

The Nutritional-Metabolic Pattern is another important component of Gordon's Functional Health Patterns, focusing on a patient's nutritional status and metabolic needs. In the context of rehabilitation nursing, evaluating the Nutritional-Metabolic Pattern is crucial for several reasons:

1. Identifying Nutritional Deficiencies: Assessing a patient's nutritional intake and status helps rehabilitation nurses identify potential deficiencies that may hinder the healing process or impact overall health. Early identification of deficiencies allows for the implementation of targeted interventions, such as dietary modifications, supplements, or referrals to nutrition specialists.
2. Monitoring Metabolic Demands: Rehabilitation often involves increased physical activity, which can lead to changes in a patient's metabolic needs. Regular evaluation of

the Nutritional-Metabolic Pattern allows nurses to ensure that patients receive adequate nutrition to support their rehabilitation goals and maintain their overall health.
3. Assessing Nutritional Risks: Certain medical conditions or treatments can put patients at risk for malnutrition or other nutritional complications. Evaluating the Nutritional-Metabolic Pattern enables rehabilitation nurses to identify patients at risk and implement appropriate interventions to minimize these risks.
4. Supporting Wound Healing: Adequate nutrition plays a vital role in the healing process, particularly for patients with wounds or surgical incisions. Assessing the Nutritional-Metabolic Pattern helps rehabilitation nurses identify nutritional needs related to wound healing and implement interventions to promote optimal recovery.
5. Promoting Long-Term Health: A balanced, nutritious diet is essential for maintaining overall health and well-being. By evaluating the Nutritional-Metabolic Pattern, rehabilitation nurses can educate patients on the importance of proper nutrition and help them develop healthy eating habits that will support their long-term health.

In summary, the Nutritional-Metabolic Pattern plays a significant role in rehabilitation nursing by helping to evaluate patients' nutritional status and metabolic needs. Assessing this pattern enables nurses to identify potential deficiencies, monitor metabolic demands, assess nutritional risks, support wound healing, and promote long-term health. This information is vital for developing individualized care plans and ensuring successful patient outcomes in the rehabilitation setting.

Elimination Pattern: Significance in Rehabilitation Nursing

The Elimination Pattern is a vital aspect of Gordon's Functional Health Patterns, focusing on a patient's bowel, bladder, and skin function. In the context of rehabilitation nursing, the Elimination Pattern plays a significant role in several ways:
1. Maintaining Comfort and Dignity: Ensuring patients' elimination needs are met and managed properly is crucial for their comfort and dignity. Rehabilitation nurses assess patients' bowel and bladder function to identify issues such as constipation, incontinence, or urinary retention and implement appropriate interventions to address these concerns.
2. Preventing Complications: Monitoring and managing elimination functions can help prevent complications such as urinary tract infections, bowel impactions, or pressure ulcers. Early identification and intervention can reduce the risk of these complications, which could otherwise hinder patients' progress in rehabilitation.
3. Supporting Independence: Many patients in rehabilitation settings aim to regain their independence in daily activities, including toileting. Assessing the Elimination Pattern allows rehabilitation nurses to determine patients' current abilities and develop individualized plans to help them achieve greater independence in managing their elimination needs.
4. Identifying Underlying Issues: Changes in a patient's elimination function can sometimes indicate an underlying medical issue. By regularly assessing the Elimination Pattern,

rehabilitation nurses can identify potential concerns and collaborate with other healthcare professionals to address these issues promptly.
5. Education and Training: An essential component of rehabilitation nursing is providing patients and their families with the necessary education and training to manage their elimination needs. This may include teaching patients about bowel and bladder health, proper techniques for using continence aids, or skin care strategies to prevent pressure ulcers.

In summary, the Elimination Pattern holds great importance in rehabilitation nursing, as it enables nurses to assess and address patients' bowel, bladder, and skin function. By focusing on elimination, nurses can maintain patient comfort and dignity, prevent complications, support independence, identify underlying issues, and provide essential education and training. Proper management of the Elimination Pattern is critical for optimizing patient outcomes in the rehabilitation setting.

Activity-Exercise Pattern: Importance in Rehabilitation Nursing

The Activity-Exercise Pattern is a key component of Gordon's Functional Health Patterns, which focuses on a patient's functional abilities, mobility, and exercise tolerance. In the context of rehabilitation nursing, the Activity-Exercise Pattern plays a critical role in several ways:

1. Assessing Functional Abilities: Rehabilitation nurses use the Activity-Exercise Pattern to evaluate a patient's current functional abilities, such as walking, transferring, or performing activities of daily living (ADLs). By understanding a patient's baseline functional status, nurses can identify areas that require improvement and set realistic goals for rehabilitation.
2. Developing Individualized Care Plans: Once a patient's functional abilities have been assessed, rehabilitation nurses can develop tailored care plans that address specific needs and goals. These care plans may include interventions such as mobility training, strength-building exercises, or adaptations to help patients perform ADLs more independently.
3. Monitoring Progress: Regularly evaluating the Activity-Exercise Pattern allows rehabilitation nurses to track a patient's progress throughout their rehabilitation journey. This ongoing assessment ensures that interventions remain effective and are adjusted as needed to promote optimal outcomes.
4. Promoting Safe Mobility: Assessing a patient's mobility is crucial for ensuring their safety in the rehabilitation setting. Rehabilitation nurses can identify potential risks, such as falls or injury, and implement preventive measures, such as providing appropriate assistive devices or ensuring a safe environment.
5. Encouraging Exercise and Physical Activity: Exercise tolerance and physical activity play a significant role in a patient's overall health and well-being. Rehabilitation nurses use the Activity-Exercise Pattern to determine a patient's exercise tolerance and develop appropriate exercise programs to improve their cardiovascular fitness, strength, and endurance.

6. Interdisciplinary Collaboration: The Activity-Exercise Pattern enables rehabilitation nurses to collaborate effectively with other healthcare professionals, such as physical therapists, occupational therapists, and physicians. This collaboration ensures that patients receive a comprehensive and coordinated approach to their rehabilitation.

In conclusion, the Activity-Exercise Pattern is essential in rehabilitation nursing, as it helps assess and address patients' functional abilities, mobility, and exercise tolerance. By focusing on the Activity-Exercise Pattern, nurses can develop individualized care plans, monitor progress, promote safe mobility, encourage physical activity, and collaborate with other healthcare professionals to optimize patient outcomes in the rehabilitation setting.

Sleep-Rest Pattern: Relevance in Rehabilitation Nursing

The Sleep-Rest Pattern is a vital component of Gordon's Functional Health Patterns, focusing on a patient's sleep quality, rest habits, and overall energy levels. In the context of rehabilitation nursing, the Sleep-Rest Pattern plays a significant role in several ways:

1. Assessing Sleep Quality: Rehabilitation nurses use the Sleep-Rest Pattern to evaluate a patient's sleep patterns, duration, and quality. Poor sleep quality can negatively impact a patient's recovery process, mood, and ability to participate in therapeutic interventions.
2. Identifying Sleep Disturbances: Assessing the Sleep-Rest Pattern helps rehabilitation nurses identify any sleep disturbances a patient may be experiencing, such as insomnia, sleep apnea, or restless leg syndrome. Early identification of these issues enables timely intervention and appropriate referrals to specialists when necessary.
3. Developing Individualized Care Plans: Once a patient's sleep and rest habits have been assessed, rehabilitation nurses can develop tailored care plans that address specific sleep-related needs. Interventions may include sleep hygiene education, relaxation techniques, or adjustments to the patient's environment to promote restful sleep.
4. Monitoring Energy Levels: Regularly evaluating the Sleep-Rest Pattern allows rehabilitation nurses to track a patient's energy levels throughout their rehabilitation journey. Low energy levels can hinder a patient's ability to engage in therapy and other activities, so it's essential to address any contributing factors.
5. Promoting Rest and Recovery: Adequate rest is crucial for patients in rehabilitation, as it allows the body to recover and heal. Rehabilitation nurses can use the Sleep-Rest Pattern to ensure patients have opportunities for rest throughout the day and implement strategies to help them conserve energy.
6. Interdisciplinary Collaboration: The Sleep-Rest Pattern enables rehabilitation nurses to collaborate effectively with other healthcare professionals, such as physicians, occupational therapists, and psychologists. This collaboration ensures that patients receive a comprehensive and coordinated approach to managing their sleep and rest needs.

In conclusion, the Sleep-Rest Pattern is essential in rehabilitation nursing, as it helps assess and address patients' sleep quality, rest habits, and overall energy levels. By focusing on the Sleep-Rest Pattern, nurses can develop individualized care plans, monitor energy levels, promote rest and recovery, and collaborate with other healthcare professionals to optimize patient outcomes in the rehabilitation setting.

Cognitive-Perceptual Pattern: Role in Rehabilitation Nursing

The Cognitive-Perceptual Pattern is a critical aspect of Gordon's Functional Health Patterns, focusing on a patient's cognitive abilities, sensory-perceptual function, and communication skills. In the context of rehabilitation nursing, the Cognitive-Perceptual Pattern plays a crucial role in several ways:

1. Assessing Cognitive Abilities: Rehabilitation nurses use the Cognitive-Perceptual Pattern to evaluate a patient's memory, attention, problem-solving skills, and overall cognitive function. This assessment helps identify any cognitive impairments that may impact the patient's rehabilitation process and their ability to perform daily activities.
2. Evaluating Sensory-Perceptual Function: The Cognitive-Perceptual Pattern enables rehabilitation nurses to assess a patient's sensory-perceptual function, including vision, hearing, touch, taste, and smell. Identifying sensory deficits allows for the implementation of appropriate interventions and accommodations to support the patient's rehabilitation journey.
3. Assessing Communication Skills: The Cognitive-Perceptual Pattern guides rehabilitation nurses in evaluating a patient's verbal and non-verbal communication skills. This assessment is crucial in determining the patient's ability to express their needs, understand instructions, and participate effectively in therapy sessions.
4. Developing Individualized Care Plans: Once a patient's cognitive-perceptual function has been assessed, rehabilitation nurses can develop tailored care plans to address specific needs. Interventions may include cognitive training, sensory stimulation, or communication strategies to enhance the patient's function and independence.
5. Monitoring Progress: Rehabilitation nurses regularly evaluate the Cognitive-Perceptual Pattern to track a patient's progress in cognitive function, sensory-perceptual abilities, and communication skills. This ongoing assessment helps identify areas of improvement and adjust care plans as needed.
6. Interdisciplinary Collaboration: The Cognitive-Perceptual Pattern supports effective collaboration with other healthcare professionals, such as speech therapists, occupational therapists, and neuropsychologists. This interdisciplinary approach ensures that patients receive comprehensive and coordinated care to address their cognitive and sensory-perceptual needs.

In conclusion, the Cognitive-Perceptual Pattern is essential in rehabilitation nursing, as it helps assess and address a patient's cognitive abilities, sensory-perceptual function, and communication skills. By focusing on the Cognitive-Perceptual Pattern, nurses can develop individualized care plans, monitor progress, and collaborate with other healthcare professionals to optimize patient outcomes in the rehabilitation setting.

Self-Perception-Self-Concept Pattern: Importance in Rehabilitation Nursing

The Self-Perception-Self-Concept Pattern is an integral aspect of Gordon's Functional Health Patterns, focusing on a patient's self-image, self-esteem, and emotional well-being. In the context of rehabilitation nursing, the Self-Perception-Self-Concept Pattern plays a vital role in several ways:

1. Assessing Self-Image and Self-Esteem: Rehabilitation nurses use the Self-Perception-Self-Concept Pattern to evaluate a patient's perception of their physical appearance, abilities, and overall worth. Understanding a patient's self-image and self-esteem is crucial in identifying potential barriers to their rehabilitation progress, as these factors can significantly impact motivation, adherence to therapy, and overall recovery.
2. Evaluating Emotional Well-being: The Self-Perception-Self-Concept Pattern enables rehabilitation nurses to assess a patient's emotional well-being, including their ability to cope with stress, express emotions, and maintain a positive outlook. Emotional well-being plays a critical role in a patient's resilience and adaptability during the rehabilitation process.
3. Developing Individualized Care Plans: Once a patient's self-perception, self-concept, and emotional well-being have been assessed, rehabilitation nurses can develop tailored care plans to address specific needs. Interventions may include emotional support, counseling, or stress management techniques to enhance the patient's psychological health and overall quality of life.
4. Monitoring Progress: Rehabilitation nurses regularly evaluate the Self-Perception-Self-Concept Pattern to track a patient's progress in self-esteem, self-image, and emotional well-being. This ongoing assessment helps identify areas of improvement and adjust care plans as needed.
5. Interdisciplinary Collaboration: The Self-Perception-Self-Concept Pattern supports effective collaboration with other healthcare professionals, such as psychologists, social workers, and occupational therapists. This interdisciplinary approach ensures that patients receive comprehensive and coordinated care to address their emotional and psychological needs.
6. Facilitating Patient Empowerment: By addressing the Self-Perception-Self-Concept Pattern, rehabilitation nurses can help patients build self-confidence, develop a sense of control, and foster a positive attitude towards their recovery. This empowerment ultimately promotes active participation and engagement in the rehabilitation process, leading to improved outcomes.

In conclusion, the Self-Perception-Self-Concept Pattern is essential in rehabilitation nursing, as it helps assess and address a patient's self-image, self-esteem, and emotional well-being. By focusing on the Self-Perception-Self-Concept Pattern, nurses can develop individualized care plans, monitor progress, and collaborate with other healthcare professionals to optimize patient outcomes in the rehabilitation setting.

Roles-Relationships Pattern: Significance in Rehabilitation Nursing

The Roles-Relationships Pattern is a crucial aspect of Gordon's Functional Health Patterns, focusing on a patient's social functioning, support systems, and their ability to maintain or adapt to their roles. In rehabilitation nursing, the Roles-Relationships Pattern is significant in several ways:

1. Assessing Social Functioning: Rehabilitation nurses use the Roles-Relationships Pattern to evaluate a patient's ability to interact with others, maintain meaningful relationships, and participate in social activities. This assessment helps identify potential challenges and barriers to social reintegration, which may impact the patient's overall recovery and quality of life.
2. Identifying Support Systems: The Roles-Relationships Pattern enables nurses to determine the strength and availability of a patient's support system, including family, friends, and community resources. A strong support system plays a vital role in promoting patient adherence to therapy, providing emotional support, and facilitating a smoother transition to daily life.
3. Evaluating Role Adaptation: Rehabilitation nursing involves assessing a patient's capacity to maintain or adapt to their roles, such as being a parent, spouse, employee, or community member. Understanding a patient's ability to fulfill these roles is essential for tailoring interventions that foster role adaptation and promote independence.
4. Developing Individualized Care Plans: Once a patient's social functioning, support systems, and role adaptation have been assessed, rehabilitation nurses can develop targeted care plans to address specific needs. Interventions may include social skills training, family counseling, or support group referrals to enhance the patient's social well-being.
5. Monitoring Progress: Rehabilitation nurses regularly evaluate the Roles-Relationships Pattern to track a patient's progress in social functioning, support system utilization, and role adaptation. This ongoing assessment helps identify areas of improvement and adjust care plans as needed.
6. Interdisciplinary Collaboration: The Roles-Relationships Pattern supports effective collaboration with other healthcare professionals, such as social workers, occupational therapists, and psychologists. This interdisciplinary approach ensures that patients receive comprehensive and coordinated care to address their social and role-related needs.

In conclusion, the Roles-Relationships Pattern is essential in rehabilitation nursing, as it helps assess and address a patient's social functioning, support systems, and ability to maintain or adapt to their roles. By focusing on the Roles-Relationships Pattern, nurses can develop individualized care plans, monitor progress, and collaborate with other healthcare professionals to optimize patient outcomes in the rehabilitation setting.

Sexuality-Reproductive Pattern: Relevance in Rehabilitation Nursing

The Sexuality-Reproductive Pattern is another essential aspect of Gordon's Functional Health Patterns, focusing on a patient's sexual health, reproductive function, and related experiences. In rehabilitation nursing, the Sexuality-Reproductive Pattern is relevant for several reasons:

Assessing Sexual Health: Rehabilitation nurses use the Sexuality-Reproductive Pattern to evaluate a patient's sexual health, including their sexual functioning, satisfaction, and any concerns or difficulties they may be experiencing. This assessment helps identify potential issues that may impact the patient's overall well-being and quality of life.

Addressing Reproductive Function: The Sexuality-Reproductive Pattern enables nurses to assess a patient's reproductive function, such as menstrual cycles, fertility, and menopause. In the context of rehabilitation, understanding a patient's reproductive function is essential for addressing any potential complications, providing appropriate education, and tailoring interventions to meet their needs.

Coping with Changes in Sexual Function: Patients undergoing rehabilitation may experience changes in their sexual function due to physical limitations, emotional distress, or side effects of medications. By evaluating the Sexuality-Reproductive Pattern, rehabilitation nurses can provide support and guidance to help patients and their partners cope with these changes and maintain a satisfying sexual relationship.

Providing Education and Resources: Assessing the Sexuality-Reproductive Pattern allows rehabilitation nurses to identify gaps in a patient's knowledge about sexual health and reproductive function. Nurses can then provide education, resources, and referrals to help patients make informed decisions and maintain optimal sexual and reproductive health.

Developing Individualized Care Plans: Once a patient's sexual health and reproductive function have been assessed, rehabilitation nurses can develop targeted care plans that address specific needs. Interventions may include counseling, physical therapy, or referral to specialized services such as fertility clinics or support groups.

Interdisciplinary Collaboration: The Sexuality-Reproductive Pattern supports effective collaboration with other healthcare professionals, such as physicians, physical therapists, and psychologists. This interdisciplinary approach ensures that patients receive comprehensive and coordinated care to address their sexual and reproductive health needs.

In conclusion, the Sexuality-Reproductive Pattern is vital in rehabilitation nursing, as it helps assess and address a patient's sexual health and reproductive function. By focusing on the Sexuality-Reproductive Pattern, nurses can develop individualized care plans, provide education and resources, and collaborate with other healthcare professionals to optimize patient outcomes in the rehabilitation setting.

Coping-Stress Tolerance Pattern: Importance in Rehabilitation Setting

The Coping-Stress Tolerance Pattern is a vital aspect of Gordon's Functional Health Patterns, focusing on a patient's ability to manage stress, cope with challenges, and demonstrate psychological resilience. In the rehabilitation setting, understanding the Coping-Stress Tolerance Pattern is essential for several reasons:

1. Identifying Coping Strategies: By evaluating the Coping-Stress Tolerance Pattern, rehabilitation nurses can identify the coping strategies patients use to handle stressors and adapt to changes in their health status. This information helps nurses determine the effectiveness of these strategies and offer guidance to enhance patients' coping skills.
2. Evaluating Stress Tolerance: Assessing the Coping-Stress Tolerance Pattern enables nurses to evaluate a patient's stress tolerance, which is their ability to withstand and recover from stressors. This assessment is crucial in understanding how well patients can manage stress during the rehabilitation process and identify any potential barriers to recovery.
3. Enhancing Psychological Resilience: Psychological resilience is a patient's ability to bounce back from adversity and maintain well-being despite challenges. By understanding the Coping-Stress Tolerance Pattern, rehabilitation nurses can develop interventions to foster psychological resilience, enabling patients to better adapt to their circumstances and continue working towards their rehabilitation goals.
4. Addressing Emotional Needs: An evaluation of the Coping-Stress Tolerance Pattern helps rehabilitation nurses identify a patient's emotional needs, including any feelings of anxiety, depression, or frustration. Nurses can then provide support, counseling, and resources to help patients manage their emotions effectively and improve their mental health.
5. Tailoring Care Plans: Once a patient's coping strategies and stress tolerance are assessed, rehabilitation nurses can develop individualized care plans that address their specific needs. Interventions may include stress management techniques, relaxation exercises, or referrals to mental health professionals.
6. Interprofessional Collaboration: Understanding the Coping-Stress Tolerance Pattern fosters collaboration with other healthcare professionals, such as psychologists, social workers, and occupational therapists. This interdisciplinary approach ensures that patients receive comprehensive care to address their psychological well-being and enhance their ability to cope with stress.

In summary, the Coping-Stress Tolerance Pattern is crucial in rehabilitation nursing, as it helps assess a patient's coping strategies, stress tolerance, and psychological resilience. By focusing on this pattern, nurses can develop targeted care plans, provide emotional support, and collaborate with other healthcare professionals to improve patient outcomes in the rehabilitation setting.

Value-Belief Pattern: Role in Rehabilitation Experience

The Value-Belief Pattern is an essential component of Gordon's Functional Health Patterns, as it helps rehabilitation nurses understand a patient's cultural, spiritual, and personal values and beliefs that may influence their rehabilitation journey. The importance of addressing the Value-Belief Pattern lies in the following aspects:

1. Individualized Care: Recognizing a patient's values and beliefs allows rehabilitation nurses to provide individualized care that respects and accommodates their unique perspectives. This approach promotes patient-centered care, leading to improved patient satisfaction and outcomes.
2. Cultural Sensitivity: Understanding a patient's cultural background and values helps nurses approach care with cultural sensitivity. By doing so, they can foster a trusting relationship with the patient and avoid potential misunderstandings or conflicts that may arise from cultural differences.
3. Spiritual Needs: Assessing the Value-Belief Pattern enables rehabilitation nurses to identify a patient's spiritual needs, which can significantly impact their overall well-being and recovery. By addressing these needs, nurses can provide holistic care that supports the patient's emotional, mental, and spiritual health.
4. Informed Decision-Making: Knowledge of a patient's values and beliefs can help rehabilitation nurses better understand their preferences and priorities, which is crucial for informed decision-making. By incorporating these insights, nurses can develop care plans that are aligned with the patient's goals and values.
5. Coping and Resilience: A patient's values and beliefs can influence their coping strategies and resilience during the rehabilitation process. By understanding the Value-Belief Pattern, nurses can support and reinforce positive coping mechanisms that align with the patient's belief system, ultimately enhancing their ability to adapt to challenges.
6. Interprofessional Collaboration: Awareness of a patient's values and beliefs facilitates collaboration with other healthcare professionals, such as chaplains, social workers, and cultural liaisons. This interdisciplinary approach ensures that patients receive comprehensive care that addresses their diverse needs and respects their values.

In conclusion, the Value-Belief Pattern plays a vital role in understanding a patient's cultural, spiritual, and personal values and beliefs that may influence their rehabilitation experience. By addressing this pattern, rehabilitation nurses can provide individualized, culturally sensitive, and holistic care that supports the patient's overall well-being and promotes positive outcomes.

Applying Functional Health Patterns in Rehabilitation Nursing Practice: Examples and Case Studies

Example 1: Stroke Rehabilitation

John, a 68-year-old man, was admitted to a rehabilitation facility following a stroke that affected his left side. The rehabilitation nurse uses Gordon's Functional Health Patterns to assess John and develop an individualized care plan.

- Health Perception-Health Management: John understands the importance of rehabilitation and is committed to following his care plan. The nurse ensures John receives education on stroke prevention and self-care strategies.
- Nutritional-Metabolic: The nurse assesses John's nutritional needs, considering his difficulty swallowing. They collaborate with a dietitian to develop a modified diet plan to ensure adequate nutrition.

- Elimination: John has occasional urinary incontinence. The nurse implements a toileting schedule and bladder training program to improve continence.
- Activity-Exercise: The nurse works with physical and occupational therapists to create an exercise program that addresses John's mobility and functional limitations.
- Sleep-Rest: John reports difficulty sleeping at night. The nurse establishes a bedtime routine and modifies the environment to promote restful sleep.
- Cognitive-Perceptual: The nurse assesses John's cognitive and communication abilities and collaborates with a speech therapist to address any deficits.
- Self-Perception-Self-Concept: John expresses frustration with his current limitations. The nurse provides emotional support and encourages John to focus on his progress and achievements.
- Roles-Relationships: The nurse involves John's family in his care, providing education and support to help them adjust to his changing needs.
- Sexuality-Reproductive: The nurse addresses any concerns John may have about intimacy and provides education on safe sexual practices.
- Coping-Stress Tolerance: The nurse assesses John's coping strategies and provides resources to help manage stress, such as relaxation techniques and support groups.
- Value-Belief: John finds solace in prayer. The nurse respects his beliefs and ensures he has the opportunity to engage in spiritual practices.

Example 2: Spinal Cord Injury Rehabilitation

Maria, a 32-year-old woman, sustained a spinal cord injury in a car accident that resulted in paraplegia. The rehabilitation nurse uses Gordon's Functional Health Patterns to assess Maria and develop an individualized care plan.

- Health Perception-Health Management: The nurse educates Maria on her injury and the importance of adhering to her rehabilitation plan. They discuss strategies to prevent complications and promote self-care.
- Nutritional-Metabolic: Maria's nutritional needs are assessed, and the nurse works with a dietitian to develop a meal plan that promotes healing and prevents pressure ulcers.
- Elimination: Maria requires assistance with bowel and bladder management. The nurse establishes a routine and teaches Maria and her family the necessary techniques.
- Activity-Exercise: The nurse collaborates with physical and occupational therapists to design a program that focuses on Maria's strength, mobility, and independence in daily activities.
- Sleep-Rest: Maria experiences pain and discomfort that disrupt her sleep. The nurse administers prescribed pain medication and employs non-pharmacological interventions to improve sleep quality.
- Cognitive-Perceptual: The nurse assesses Maria's cognitive function and ensures she is provided with any necessary assistive devices for communication.
- Self-Perception-Self-Concept: Maria struggles with her new physical limitations and the impact on her self-esteem. The nurse offers emotional support and encourages Maria to join a support group for individuals with spinal cord injuries.

- Roles-Relationships: The nurse involves Maria's family in her care and provides education on adapting to her new needs and maintaining supportive relationships.
- Sexuality-Reproductive: The nurse addresses Maria's concerns about her sexual health and provides education on maintaining a fulfilling sexual relationship.
- Coping-Stress Tolerance: The nurse assesses Maria's coping mechanisms and stress tolerance, providing her with resources such as relaxation techniques, counseling, and peer support groups to help her navigate this challenging time.
- Value-Belief: Maria identifies as a spiritual person, finding comfort in meditation and mindfulness practices. The nurse ensures Maria has the opportunity to engage in these activities to support her emotional well-being.
- Through these two case studies, we can see how rehabilitation nurses can effectively apply Gordon's Functional Health Patterns to assess patients holistically, develop individualized care plans, and monitor progress throughout the rehabilitation process. By addressing each aspect of a patient's health and well-being, rehabilitation nurses can help patients adapt to their new circumstances, prevent complications, and ultimately, improve their quality of life

In this chapter, we explored the concept of functional health patterns and their vital role in rehabilitation nursing. We delved into Marjory Gordon's Functional Health Patterns framework, discussing each of the 11 patterns and their significance in assessing and addressing a patient's needs comprehensively. We highlighted the importance of evaluating patients' understanding of their health, nutritional status, functional abilities, sleep quality, cognitive abilities, self-image, social functioning, sexual health, coping strategies, and cultural, spiritual, and personal values.

Using case studies, we illustrated how rehabilitation nurses can employ functional health patterns to develop individualized care plans, monitor progress, and adapt their interventions to meet patients' changing needs. By integrating this holistic approach into their practice, rehabilitation nurses can better understand their patients' unique circumstances, implement evidence-based interventions, and ultimately, enhance patient outcomes.

In conclusion, functional health patterns offer a valuable framework for rehabilitation nursing practice, allowing professionals to provide comprehensive, patient-centered care that addresses the complex and interrelated aspects of a patient's health and well-being. By consistently applying these patterns, rehabilitation nurses can contribute to the ongoing improvement of patient outcomes and advance the profession as a whole.

The Rehabilitation Nursing Process

The Rehabilitation Nursing Process is a systematic, organized method used by rehabilitation nurses to provide patient-centered care, focusing on the unique needs of individuals recovering from illness, injury, or surgery. It is an essential framework that guides rehabilitation nurses in assessing, diagnosing, planning, implementing, and evaluating patient care to facilitate optimal outcomes and enhance patients' quality of life.

The core components of the Rehabilitation Nursing Process include:

1. Assessment: This involves collecting comprehensive information about a patient's health status, functional abilities, and personal needs. Rehabilitation nurses gather data through patient interviews, physical examinations, medical history reviews, and consultations with other healthcare professionals.
2. Diagnosis: Based on the assessment findings, rehabilitation nurses identify actual or potential health problems, functional limitations, and patient concerns. They formulate nursing diagnoses that guide the development of individualized care plans.
3. Planning: In this step, rehabilitation nurses collaborate with patients, their families, and interdisciplinary team members to set realistic, measurable, and patient-centered goals. They develop care plans that outline specific interventions and strategies to address each nursing diagnosis.
4. Implementation: Rehabilitation nurses carry out the interventions outlined in the care plan, adapting their approach as needed to meet patients' unique needs and preferences. They also engage patients and their families in the care process, empowering them to take an active role in their recovery.
5. Evaluation: The rehabilitation nursing process involves ongoing evaluation of patients' progress toward their goals. Nurses reassess patients' needs, monitor the effectiveness of interventions, and adjust care plans as necessary to ensure optimal outcomes.

The Rehabilitation Nursing Process is crucial in the rehabilitation setting, as it ensures that care is tailored to patients' individual needs and goals, promoting their physical, emotional, and social well-being. By following this structured approach, rehabilitation nurses can provide high-quality care that supports patients throughout their recovery journey, ultimately helping them achieve the best possible outcomes and enhancing their quality of life.

Assessment is a vital component of the rehabilitation nursing process, as it lays the foundation for developing individualized care plans that address patients' unique needs and goals. The primary purpose of assessment in rehabilitation nursing is to gather comprehensive information about a patient's health status, functional abilities, and personal preferences, which allows nurses to tailor their approach and ensure the best possible outcomes.

The assessment process involves multiple steps:

1. Collecting information: Rehabilitation nurses gather data through patient interviews, physical examinations, medical history reviews, and consultations with other healthcare professionals. This information provides valuable insights into the patient's physical, emotional, and social needs, as well as their expectations and concerns.

2. Using standardized assessment tools: To ensure consistency and accuracy, rehabilitation nurses often use standardized assessment tools when evaluating patients. These tools may assess various aspects of a patient's health and function, such as mobility, strength, balance, and cognition. They provide objective data that help nurses identify areas requiring intervention and track progress over time.
3. Identifying individual needs and goals: During the assessment process, rehabilitation nurses also identify patients' unique needs and goals, which may include returning to work, regaining independence, or improving their quality of life. By understanding patients' individual priorities and aspirations, nurses can better tailor their care plans and interventions to support patients in achieving their desired outcomes.

In conclusion, assessment is a critical aspect of the rehabilitation nursing process that helps nurses understand patients' unique needs and goals. By gathering comprehensive information, using standardized assessment tools, and focusing on patients' individual priorities, rehabilitation nurses can develop care plans that optimize patient outcomes and enhance their overall well-being.

Diagnosis in rehabilitation nursing is a crucial step in the nursing process, as it helps identify specific patient concerns and develop targeted interventions to address them. Formulating accurate nursing diagnoses in the context of rehabilitation involves analyzing the assessment data, prioritizing patient concerns, and collaborating with the interdisciplinary team to ensure a comprehensive approach to patient care.

1. Analyzing assessment data: After gathering comprehensive information about the patient's health status, functional abilities, and personal preferences, rehabilitation nurses analyze this data to identify patterns and trends. This analysis helps nurses pinpoint areas that require intervention and develop nursing diagnoses based on the patient's needs.
2. Accurate diagnosis: Formulating accurate nursing diagnoses is essential, as it guides the development of individualized care plans and interventions. Rehabilitation nurses use standardized nursing language and classification systems, such as the NANDA International (NANDA-I) taxonomy, to ensure consistency and clarity in their diagnoses. Accurate diagnosis also enables better communication among healthcare professionals and facilitates the evaluation of care outcomes.
3. Prioritizing patient concerns: In the diagnosis phase, rehabilitation nurses must prioritize patient concerns to focus on the most pressing issues first. This prioritization process considers the patient's preferences, the severity of their concerns, and the potential impact on their overall well-being. By addressing the most critical issues first, nurses can optimize their interventions and maximize patient outcomes.
4. Interdisciplinary collaboration: Rehabilitation nursing often involves working with an interdisciplinary team of healthcare professionals, such as physicians, therapists, and social workers. This collaboration is essential when formulating nursing diagnoses, as it ensures that all aspects of a patient's care are considered and that potential gaps in care

are addressed. Effective communication and collaboration among team members can lead to more accurate diagnoses and better overall care.

In summary, the process of formulating nursing diagnoses in rehabilitation nursing involves analyzing assessment data, ensuring accurate diagnoses, prioritizing patient concerns, and incorporating interdisciplinary collaboration. This process is essential for developing individualized care plans and interventions that effectively address patients' needs and help them achieve their rehabilitation goals.

Planning in rehabilitation nursing is a vital component of the nursing process, as it involves developing individualized care plans tailored to each patient's unique needs and goals. The process of planning in rehabilitation nursing focuses on setting realistic, measurable, and patient-centered goals while emphasizing the role of interdisciplinary teamwork.

1. Setting realistic goals: When developing care plans, rehabilitation nurses work closely with patients to establish achievable goals. These goals should take into account the patient's current health status, functional abilities, and personal preferences, ensuring that the objectives are both realistic and meaningful to the patient.
2. Measurable goals: In addition to being realistic, goals must also be measurable, allowing nurses to monitor progress and adjust interventions as needed. Measurable goals include specific criteria that can be evaluated, such as the level of pain relief, the degree of functional improvement, or the timeframe for achieving a particular outcome.
3. Patient-centered goals: The planning process in rehabilitation nursing is patient-centered, meaning that the goals and interventions are aligned with the patient's preferences and values. By involving patients in the decision-making process and respecting their autonomy, rehabilitation nurses can create care plans that are truly tailored to the individual's needs and desires.
4. Interdisciplinary teamwork: Effective planning in rehabilitation nursing requires close collaboration among an interdisciplinary team of healthcare professionals, such as physicians, therapists, and social workers. This teamwork ensures that the care plan addresses all aspects of the patient's rehabilitation journey, from physical and emotional well-being to social support and environmental factors. Interdisciplinary collaboration also helps to identify and address any potential gaps in care or resources that may impact the patient's progress.

In summary, the planning process in rehabilitation nursing involves developing individualized care plans by setting realistic, measurable, and patient-centered goals while engaging in interdisciplinary teamwork. This approach ensures that patients receive comprehensive, tailored care that effectively addresses their needs and supports their rehabilitation journey.

Implementation in rehabilitation nursing is a crucial step in the nursing process, as it involves putting the carefully developed care plans into action. This step entails selecting evidence-based interventions, tailoring care to the individual needs of patients, and actively engaging both patients and their families in the care process.

1. Selecting evidence-based interventions: Rehabilitation nurses must utilize current research and best practices to identify the most effective interventions for their patients. Evidence-based interventions are those that have been shown through rigorous research to improve patient outcomes. By implementing these interventions, rehabilitation nurses can ensure that they are providing the highest quality care possible to promote recovery and well-being.
2. Tailoring care to patients' needs: Implementation in rehabilitation nursing requires adapting interventions to meet the unique needs and preferences of each patient. This may involve modifying techniques, adjusting the intensity or frequency of interventions, or incorporating alternative approaches to address specific challenges or barriers. By individualizing care, rehabilitation nurses can optimize the effectiveness of interventions and promote patient engagement and satisfaction.
3. Engaging patients and their families in the care process: An essential aspect of implementation in rehabilitation nursing is actively involving patients and their families in the care process. This includes educating them about their condition, treatment options, and self-care strategies, as well as encouraging them to participate in decision-making and goal-setting. Engaging patients and families in this manner not only fosters a sense of ownership and empowerment but also improves adherence to treatment plans and enhances overall outcomes.

In conclusion, implementation in the rehabilitation nursing process involves selecting evidence-based interventions, tailoring care to patients' unique needs, and actively engaging patients and their families in the care process. By taking these steps, rehabilitation nurses can ensure that they are providing high-quality, personalized care that promotes optimal recovery and well-being for their patients.

Evaluation is a vital component of the rehabilitation nursing process, as it involves continuously monitoring patient progress, reassessing goals, and adjusting care plans as needed. This ongoing evaluation ensures that the care provided remains effective and responsive to the patient's changing needs and circumstances.

1. Monitoring patient progress: Regularly evaluating patient progress is essential for gauging the effectiveness of interventions and determining whether patients are moving towards their established goals. Rehabilitation nurses must closely observe and document changes in patients' functional abilities, symptoms, and overall well-being to identify areas of improvement, as well as any potential setbacks or complications.
2. Reassessing goals: As patients progress through their rehabilitation journey, their needs and priorities may change. Consequently, it is crucial for rehabilitation nurses to reassess goals periodically, ensuring that they remain relevant, achievable, and aligned with patients' current needs and preferences. This reassessment may involve revising existing goals, setting new ones, or even removing goals that have become obsolete or unattainable.
3. Adjusting care plans as needed: The dynamic nature of rehabilitation nursing requires that care plans be flexible and adaptive. Based on the findings from ongoing

evaluations, rehabilitation nurses may need to modify care plans to address any unanticipated issues, capitalize on emerging opportunities for improvement, or accommodate changes in patients' needs or goals. Adjusting care plans in response to evaluations ensures that care remains targeted and effective, promoting optimal patient outcomes.

In summary, ongoing evaluation is a critical aspect of the rehabilitation nursing process. By diligently monitoring patient progress, reassessing goals, and adjusting care plans as needed, rehabilitation nurses can ensure that their care remains patient-centered, effective, and responsive to the ever-evolving needs of the individuals they serve. This ongoing evaluation process is crucial for achieving optimal patient outcomes and fostering successful rehabilitation journeys.

Thorough documentation and effective communication are essential components of the rehabilitation nursing process, as they play a pivotal role in ensuring continuity of care and optimal patient outcomes. Accurate record-keeping and interdisciplinary collaboration contribute significantly to the overall success of rehabilitation efforts.

1. Accurate record-keeping: Meticulous documentation of patient assessments, care plans, interventions, and progress updates allows rehabilitation nurses to track changes in patients' conditions, identify trends, and make informed decisions about their care. Well-organized and up-to-date patient records facilitate smooth transitions between different care providers, reducing the risk of errors or miscommunication that could negatively impact patient outcomes. Furthermore, accurate documentation can serve as a valuable resource for evaluating the effectiveness of specific interventions and informing future practice.

2. Interdisciplinary collaboration: Rehabilitation is often a complex and multifaceted process, requiring the expertise of various healthcare professionals. Effective communication between team members is crucial to ensure a coordinated and comprehensive approach to patient care. By sharing information, insights, and updates with other members of the interdisciplinary team, rehabilitation nurses help to create a seamless, integrated care experience that addresses all aspects of a patient's needs. This collaborative approach contributes to better patient outcomes, as it enables the team to develop and implement more effective, patient-centered care plans.

3. Ensuring continuity of care: Thorough documentation and effective communication play a vital role in maintaining continuity of care throughout the rehabilitation process. By maintaining accurate, up-to-date records and actively engaging in interdisciplinary collaboration, rehabilitation nurses can ensure that care transitions are smooth and that all members of the healthcare team have access to the information they need to provide effective, coordinated care. This continuity is crucial for preventing gaps in care, reducing the risk of complications, and promoting a more positive rehabilitation experience for patients and their families.

In conclusion, thorough documentation and effective communication are integral to the rehabilitation nursing process. By emphasizing accurate record-keeping and interdisciplinary collaboration, rehabilitation nurses can ensure continuity of care, promote a coordinated approach to treatment, and ultimately contribute to improved patient outcomes in the rehabilitation setting.

Ethical considerations are fundamental to the rehabilitation nursing process, as they guide the decision-making and actions of healthcare professionals in their pursuit of providing optimal patient care. Four core ethical principles—patient autonomy, beneficence, non-maleficence, and justice—serve as the foundation for ethical conduct in rehabilitation nursing.

1. Patient Autonomy: This principle emphasizes the importance of respecting patients' rights to make informed decisions about their care. Rehabilitation nurses should provide patients with the necessary information, support, and encouragement to make choices that align with their values, preferences, and goals. This involves fostering an open dialogue, ensuring patients understand their options, and respecting their decisions, even if they differ from the healthcare professional's perspective.
2. Beneficence: Beneficence is the ethical obligation to promote the well-being and best interests of patients. Rehabilitation nurses should strive to provide care that maximizes patients' potential for recovery, independence, and quality of life. This involves staying up to date on evidence-based practices, tailoring interventions to individual needs, and advocating for patients' needs within the interdisciplinary team.
3. Non-maleficence: This principle highlights the need to avoid causing harm or suffering to patients. Rehabilitation nurses must carefully consider the potential risks and benefits of interventions, striving to minimize harm while promoting positive outcomes. This may involve close monitoring of patients' responses to interventions, adjusting care plans as needed, and discontinuing treatments that cause undue harm or fail to provide meaningful benefits.
4. Justice: Justice in rehabilitation nursing refers to the fair and equitable distribution of resources, treatment opportunities, and respect for patients. Rehabilitation nurses should work to ensure that all patients have equal access to high-quality care, regardless of factors such as age, gender, race, or socioeconomic status. This may involve advocating for policies and practices that address disparities in healthcare and promoting a culture of inclusivity and respect within the rehabilitation setting.

In conclusion, the ethical principles of patient autonomy, beneficence, non-maleficence, and justice play a vital role in guiding the rehabilitation nursing process. By incorporating these principles into their practice, rehabilitation nurses can make informed, ethically sound decisions that prioritize patient well-being and promote the highest possible standards of care.

Cultural competence is essential in the rehabilitation nursing process, as it enables healthcare professionals to provide care that is both respectful and responsive to the diverse cultural backgrounds, beliefs, and values of patients. By developing cultural competence, rehabilitation nurses can better understand patients' unique needs, foster trusting relationships, and promote health equity. Here are some strategies for providing culturally sensitive care:

1. Self-awareness: Rehabilitation nurses should engage in self-reflection to identify their own cultural biases, beliefs, and values, which may influence their interactions with patients. By acknowledging these biases and striving to overcome them, nurses can provide care that is respectful and nonjudgmental.
2. Cultural knowledge: Healthcare professionals should strive to expand their understanding of different cultural practices, beliefs, and values that may affect patients' healthcare experiences. This can be achieved through ongoing education, training, and exposure to diverse cultural perspectives.
3. Active listening and communication: Rehabilitation nurses should use active listening and open-ended questions to elicit patients' perspectives and preferences regarding their care. By adapting communication styles and utilizing culturally appropriate language, nurses can foster an environment in which patients feel comfortable expressing their needs and concerns.
4. Patient-centered care: Nurses should collaborate with patients to develop individualized care plans that align with their cultural beliefs, values, and preferences. This may involve incorporating traditional healing practices, seeking input from family members, or providing care in a manner that is consistent with patients' cultural norms.
5. Advocacy and health equity: Rehabilitation nurses should advocate for policies and practices that promote health equity, address disparities in care, and create an inclusive environment for all patients. This may involve engaging in community outreach, supporting language services, or collaborating with interdisciplinary teams to develop culturally appropriate resources and services.

In summary, cultural competence plays a critical role in the rehabilitation nursing process. By incorporating strategies such as self-awareness, cultural knowledge, active listening, patient-centered care, and advocacy, rehabilitation nurses can provide culturally sensitive care and promote health equity for patients from diverse backgrounds. This approach helps ensure that every patient has an opportunity to achieve the best possible outcomes during their rehabilitation journey.

Interprofessional collaboration is crucial in the rehabilitation nursing process, as it brings together healthcare professionals from various disciplines to provide comprehensive, patient-centered care. This interdisciplinary approach enhances the quality of care, facilitates better patient outcomes, and promotes a more efficient use of resources. Below are some benefits of interdisciplinary teamwork and strategies for fostering effective communication and cooperation:

1. Comprehensive care: Interprofessional collaboration allows each team member to contribute their unique expertise and perspectives, resulting in a more holistic understanding of the patient's needs and goals. This enables the development of well-rounded, tailored care plans that address all aspects of the patient's rehabilitation.
2. Improved patient outcomes: Studies have shown that interprofessional collaboration can lead to better patient outcomes, including improved functional status, decreased

length of stay, and reduced healthcare costs. By working together, the team can more effectively address complex patient needs and prevent potential complications.
3. Shared decision-making: Interdisciplinary teamwork fosters a shared decision-making process that involves input from all team members, the patient, and their family. This collaborative approach ensures that care plans are based on the best available evidence, align with the patient's goals, and consider the perspectives of all involved parties.
4. Enhanced learning and professional growth: Working in an interprofessional team offers opportunities for ongoing learning and professional growth, as team members can learn from one another's expertise, share knowledge, and develop new skills. This collaborative environment fosters innovation and encourages the adoption of best practices.

Strategies for fostering effective communication and cooperation in interprofessional collaboration:
1. Establish clear roles and responsibilities: Team members should have a clear understanding of their roles and responsibilities, as well as those of their colleagues. This clarity can help prevent duplication of effort and ensure that all aspects of care are addressed.
2. Develop shared goals and objectives: Collaborative goal-setting can help align the efforts of all team members and ensure that everyone is working towards the same desired outcomes.
3. Implement regular team meetings: Regular team meetings provide a forum for discussing patient progress, reassessing goals, and addressing any challenges or barriers to care. These meetings can facilitate open communication and ensure that all team members are on the same page.
4. Promote a culture of respect and trust: Fostering a supportive, respectful, and trusting team environment is essential for effective collaboration. Encourage open communication, active listening, and constructive feedback to build trust among team members.
5. Utilize effective communication tools and strategies: Implementing standardized communication tools, such as SBAR (Situation, Background, Assessment, Recommendation), can help facilitate clear and concise information exchange between team members.

In summary, interprofessional collaboration is vital to the rehabilitation nursing process. By working together, interdisciplinary teams can provide comprehensive care, improve patient outcomes, and foster a culture of continuous learning and professional growth. Emphasizing clear communication, shared goals, and mutual respect can help strengthen collaboration and ensure optimal care for patients in rehabilitation settings.

In conclusion, the rehabilitation nursing process is an essential framework that guides patient-centered care in rehabilitation settings. The key points covered in this chapter include the core components of the process: assessment, diagnosis, planning, implementation, evaluation, documentation, and communication. We also explored ethical considerations, cultural competence, and interprofessional collaboration as vital aspects of the rehabilitation nursing process.

The process starts with a comprehensive assessment of the patient's needs and goals, which informs the formulation of accurate nursing diagnoses. Based on these diagnoses, individualized care plans are developed, incorporating realistic, measurable, and patient-centered goals. Interdisciplinary teamwork is crucial in ensuring well-rounded care plans. During the implementation phase, evidence-based interventions are selected and tailored to the patient's needs, while actively involving patients and their families in the care process.

Ongoing evaluation is essential to monitor patient progress, reassess goals, and adjust care plans as needed. Thorough documentation and effective communication play a critical role in ensuring continuity of care and facilitating interdisciplinary collaboration. The rehabilitation nursing process is underpinned by ethical principles, such as patient autonomy, beneficence, non-maleficence, and justice, which guide decision-making and promote patient-centered care.

Cultural competence is crucial to providing culturally sensitive care and promoting health equity. Interprofessional collaboration is vital to achieving optimal patient outcomes, as it brings together the expertise of various healthcare professionals and fosters effective communication and cooperation.

In summary, the rehabilitation nursing process is integral to providing patient-centered care, facilitating optimal patient outcomes, and advancing the profession of rehabilitation nursing. By adhering to this process and embracing its core components and principles, rehabilitation nurses can ensure that their patients receive the best possible care on their journey towards recovery and improved quality of life.

Community Reintegration

Community reintegration is a crucial component of the rehabilitation process, as it involves helping patients transition from a healthcare setting back into their homes and communities after experiencing illness, injury, or disability. The primary goal of community reintegration is to enable individuals to regain their independence and resume their daily activities, roles, and responsibilities to the best of their ability. This process not only enhances the quality of life for the patients but also supports their overall well-being and long-term recovery.

Rehabilitation nurses play a vital role in facilitating successful community reintegration. They work closely with patients, families, and interdisciplinary teams to develop and implement comprehensive reintegration plans tailored to each individual's unique needs and goals. These plans may encompass various aspects of a patient's life, including physical and emotional health, social support, housing, transportation, employment, and community participation.

Some key responsibilities of rehabilitation nurses in community reintegration include:

1. Assessing the patient's readiness for reintegration by evaluating their physical, cognitive, emotional, and social functioning.
2. Collaborating with interdisciplinary teams to create individualized reintegration plans that address the patient's needs and goals.
3. Providing education and support to patients and their families to prepare them for the transition and help them navigate potential challenges.
4. Coordinating with community resources and support services to ensure that patients have access to the necessary assistance and opportunities for successful reintegration.
5. Monitoring patient progress and adjusting care plans as needed to address any emerging issues or changing circumstances.

In summary, community reintegration is an essential aspect of the rehabilitation process, and rehabilitation nurses play a crucial role in helping patients make a smooth and successful transition back into their communities. By providing individualized care, support, and resources, rehabilitation nurses contribute significantly to improving patient outcomes and enhancing their overall quality of life.

Community reintegration can be a challenging process for many patients, as they face various barriers that may hinder their ability to successfully reintegrate into their daily lives. These barriers can be classified into several categories, including physical, cognitive, emotional, social, and environmental factors.

Physical barriers: Some patients may experience difficulties with mobility, strength, or endurance, which can limit their ability to perform daily tasks or participate in community activities. Additionally, chronic pain or fatigue may also impede their progress.

Cognitive barriers: Cognitive impairments, such as memory, attention, or problem-solving deficits, can make it challenging for patients to adapt to new routines, manage medications, or maintain their safety at home and in the community.

Emotional barriers: Emotional factors, including depression, anxiety, or fear, can significantly impact a patient's motivation and willingness to engage in the reintegration process. Adjusting to a new reality and coping with the loss of independence can be emotionally taxing.

Social barriers: Social isolation, stigma, or lack of support from family and friends can hinder a patient's reintegration. Social barriers may also include difficulties in rebuilding relationships or establishing new connections in the community.

Environmental barriers: Environmental factors, such as inaccessible housing, limited transportation options, or lack of available support services in the community, can create obstacles for patients trying to reintegrate. Additionally, financial constraints or limited access to healthcare resources may exacerbate these challenges.

By understanding these common barriers, rehabilitation nurses and interdisciplinary teams can develop targeted interventions and support strategies to help patients overcome these obstacles, ultimately promoting successful community reintegration. It is crucial to address each patient's unique needs and circumstances to provide the most effective and comprehensive care.

Assessing a patient's readiness for community reintegration is a crucial step in the rehabilitation process. This assessment helps rehabilitation nurses and the interdisciplinary team to determine the patient's abilities, needs, and areas that require support or intervention. To evaluate readiness, the team should consider the patient's physical, cognitive, emotional, and social functioning.

1. Physical functioning: Assess the patient's ability to perform activities of daily living (ADLs) and instrumental activities of daily living (IADLs). This includes evaluating their mobility, strength, endurance, and any specific skills required for their living environment. Occupational and physical therapists can contribute valuable insights into the patient's physical abilities and limitations.
2. Cognitive functioning: Evaluate the patient's cognitive abilities, such as memory, attention, executive function, and problem-solving skills. This assessment will help to determine whether the patient can manage medications, maintain safety at home, and adapt to new routines. Neuropsychological assessments and input from speech therapists can be particularly useful in assessing cognitive functioning.
3. Emotional functioning: Assess the patient's emotional well-being, including their ability to cope with stress, manage anxiety, and deal with any feelings of depression or fear. A mental health professional, such as a psychologist or psychiatrist, can help evaluate the patient's emotional state and identify any potential challenges that may impede their reintegration process.
4. Social functioning: Assess the patient's social support system and their ability to form and maintain relationships in the community. Consider factors such as family

involvement, friendships, and participation in social or recreational activities. A social worker or case manager can provide insights into the patient's social environment and help identify resources or support networks.

By evaluating a patient's readiness for community reintegration in these four areas, the rehabilitation team can develop a comprehensive and individualized plan that addresses the patient's needs, strengthens their abilities, and provides support in areas where they may face challenges. This approach ensures that the patient has the best possible chance of achieving a successful and fulfilling reintegration into their community.

Creating a comprehensive community reintegration plan involves a collaborative and patient-centered approach. This plan should be tailored to the individual's needs, goals, and abilities, while also considering potential barriers and available resources. The process of developing a reintegration plan involves several key steps:

1. Establish individualized goals: Begin by identifying the patient's short-term and long-term goals for reintegration. These goals should be specific, measurable, achievable, relevant, and time-bound (SMART). Encourage the patient and their family to participate in this process, as their input is invaluable in setting realistic and meaningful objectives.
2. Interdisciplinary collaboration: Involve all members of the rehabilitation team, including rehabilitation nurses, physicians, occupational therapists, physical therapists, speech therapists, psychologists, social workers, and case managers. Each team member brings unique expertise and insights that contribute to a well-rounded and effective plan.
3. Assess resources and support: Determine the resources and support systems available to the patient in their community. This may include accessible housing, transportation, healthcare services, vocational training, and recreational opportunities. Assess any gaps in resources and identify strategies to address them, such as connecting the patient with local organizations or support groups.
4. Address barriers: Identify and address any potential barriers to community reintegration, such as physical, cognitive, emotional, or social challenges. Develop strategies to help the patient overcome these obstacles, which may involve additional therapy, education, or community-based support services.
5. Patient and family involvement: Engage the patient and their family in the planning process, ensuring they understand the goals and strategies of the reintegration plan. Encourage their active participation and provide them with the necessary information and resources to support the patient's transition back into the community.
6. Monitor and adjust: Regularly review the reintegration plan and adjust it as needed based on the patient's progress, new challenges, or changes in their circumstances. Ongoing evaluation and flexibility are essential to ensure the plan remains relevant and effective in meeting the patient's needs.

By following these steps, rehabilitation nurses and the interdisciplinary team can develop a comprehensive community reintegration plan that empowers the patient to achieve their goals and return to a fulfilling and independent life within their community.

Physical and occupational therapy play vital roles in preparing patients for successful community reintegration. Both therapies focus on enhancing patients' functional abilities and quality of life, enabling them to participate in meaningful activities and become more independent within their communities. While physical therapy primarily addresses mobility and strength, occupational therapy focuses on daily activities and adaptations to optimize function.

Physical therapy in community reintegration:
1. Mobility and strength: Physical therapists help patients improve their mobility by working on gait, balance, and muscle strength. This enables patients to navigate their communities more effectively and safely, including managing curbs, stairs, and uneven surfaces.
2. Endurance: Physical therapists work on patients' endurance and cardiovascular fitness, which are essential for participating in community activities and maintaining overall health.
3. Pain management: Physical therapists develop strategies for managing chronic pain, which may otherwise impede patients' ability to engage in daily tasks and community activities.
4. Assistive devices: Physical therapists may recommend and train patients to use assistive devices, such as wheelchairs, walkers, or canes, to enhance their mobility and independence.

Occupational therapy in community reintegration:
1. Activities of daily living (ADLs): Occupational therapists help patients regain the ability to perform daily tasks, such as dressing, bathing, and meal preparation, which are crucial for independence.
2. Instrumental activities of daily living (IADLs): Occupational therapists also focus on more complex tasks, such as managing finances, grocery shopping, and using public transportation, which are essential for successful community reintegration.
3. Home and environmental modifications: Occupational therapists may assess patients' homes and recommend modifications to make them more accessible and functional, such as installing grab bars, ramps, or widening doorways.
4. Adaptive equipment: Occupational therapists can recommend and train patients to use adaptive equipment, such as dressing aids, modified utensils, or communication devices, to facilitate greater independence in daily activities.
5. Community resources: Occupational therapists can connect patients with community resources and programs, such as vocational rehabilitation, support groups, or recreational activities, to enhance their social participation and overall well-being.

Together, physical and occupational therapy provide a comprehensive approach to rehabilitation, equipping patients with the necessary skills, adaptations, and confidence to successfully reintegrate into their communities and lead fulfilling lives.

Psychosocial support and counseling are essential components in facilitating community reintegration for patients undergoing rehabilitation. Addressing emotional and mental well-

being, coping strategies, stress management, and support networks is crucial in helping patients successfully adapt to their new circumstances and thrive in their communities.
1. Coping strategies: Counseling can help patients develop effective coping strategies to manage the challenges they may face during reintegration. Techniques such as problem-solving, goal setting, and cognitive restructuring can be taught to promote resilience and empower patients to overcome obstacles.
2. Stress management: Managing stress is critical for maintaining mental health and overall well-being. Counseling can equip patients with various stress management tools, such as relaxation techniques, mindfulness, and time management, which can enhance their ability to handle daily stressors and adjust to their new environment.
3. Emotional support: Psychosocial counseling provides a safe space for patients to express their feelings, concerns, and fears related to their rehabilitation and reintegration. This emotional support is essential for validating patients' experiences and helping them process any feelings of loss, grief, or frustration they may encounter during their transition.
4. Support networks: Establishing and maintaining a robust support network is vital for successful community reintegration. Counseling can help patients identify and connect with friends, family members, and community resources that can offer practical assistance, emotional support, and companionship. This may include support groups, recreational activities, and local organizations that cater to their specific needs.
5. Building self-esteem and confidence: Psychosocial counseling can also contribute to rebuilding patients' self-esteem and confidence, which may have been affected by their injury or illness. Enhancing self-esteem can empower patients to engage in community activities and social interactions, fostering a sense of belonging and purpose.

In summary, psychosocial support and counseling play a crucial role in promoting successful community reintegration by addressing emotional and mental well-being, teaching coping strategies and stress management, and fostering strong support networks. These elements are vital for patients to adapt, thrive, and lead fulfilling lives in their communities.

Vocational rehabilitation and employment support play a pivotal role in community reintegration, as they directly contribute to an individual's sense of purpose, self-worth, and financial stability. By focusing on job training, job placement, and workplace accommodations, rehabilitation professionals can empower patients to rejoin the workforce and lead fulfilling, independent lives.
1. Job training: Vocational rehabilitation programs often provide job training to help patients develop new skills or improve existing ones to increase their employability. These trainings may include computer courses, soft skills development, trade-specific training, or educational programs tailored to the patient's unique needs and abilities. Job training can also help patients gain confidence in their abilities and better adapt to workplace demands.
2. Job placement: Employment specialists within vocational rehabilitation programs work closely with patients to identify suitable job opportunities based on their skills, interests,

and limitations. They also assist with job search strategies, resume writing, interview preparation, and networking, enabling patients to successfully navigate the job market and find appropriate positions.
3. Workplace accommodations: For patients with specific needs or disabilities, workplace accommodations are crucial in ensuring a smooth transition back to work. Vocational rehabilitation professionals can collaborate with employers to identify and implement necessary accommodations, such as modified work schedules, assistive technology, ergonomic adjustments, or task reassignments. These adjustments help create an inclusive and supportive work environment, allowing patients to perform their job duties effectively and safely.
4. Employer education and support: Vocational rehabilitation programs may also involve educating employers about the benefits of hiring individuals with disabilities and addressing any concerns or misconceptions. This can promote a more inclusive work culture, reducing stigma and fostering understanding around the unique challenges and strengths of employees with disabilities.
5. Ongoing support: Following job placement, vocational rehabilitation professionals may continue to provide ongoing support to patients, monitoring their progress, addressing any workplace challenges, and assisting with career advancement or transitions as needed.

In summary, vocational rehabilitation and employment support are vital components of community reintegration, as they contribute to a patient's sense of purpose, self-worth, and financial stability. By focusing on job training, job placement, and workplace accommodations, rehabilitation professionals can help patients successfully reintegrate into the workforce and lead fulfilling, independent lives.

Accessible housing and home modifications are crucial components of community reintegration, as they create safe and supportive living environments that enable individuals to live independently and participate fully in daily life. These modifications can significantly improve a person's quality of life, promote independence, and enhance overall well-being.
1. Accessible housing: Accessible housing refers to residential spaces designed or adapted to accommodate the specific needs of individuals with disabilities or functional limitations. Features of accessible housing may include wider doorways, ramps or lifts, lower countertops, grab bars in bathrooms, and step-free entrances. Ensuring that a patient's home is accessible can make daily tasks easier, reduce the risk of injury, and foster independence.
2. Home modifications: For patients returning to their existing homes, home modifications may be necessary to create a supportive and safe living environment. These modifications can range from simple changes, such as installing grab bars or non-slip flooring, to more extensive renovations, such as installing wheelchair ramps, widening doorways, or adding accessible bathrooms. Rehabilitation professionals can work with patients and their families to identify appropriate modifications based on the individual's unique needs and limitations.

3. Collaboration with occupational therapists: Occupational therapists play a critical role in assessing a patient's home environment and recommending modifications to improve accessibility and safety. They can provide valuable insights into the patient's functional abilities, offer guidance on suitable adaptations, and help prioritize modifications based on the individual's needs and resources.
4. Funding and resources: The process of securing accessible housing or implementing home modifications can be challenging due to financial constraints or limited availability of suitable options. Rehabilitation professionals can help patients and their families navigate funding options, such as government programs, grants, or loans, and connect them with local resources, contractors, or organizations that specialize in accessible housing and home modifications.

In summary, accessible housing and home modifications play a vital role in community reintegration by creating safe and supportive living environments that promote independence and enhance overall well-being. By ensuring that patients have access to appropriate housing and necessary modifications, rehabilitation professionals can significantly improve their patients' quality of life and facilitate successful reintegration into the community.

Community resources and support services are essential components of the reintegration process, as they provide patients and their families with access to various forms of assistance, information, and opportunities for social engagement. These resources can help individuals adapt to their new circumstances, maintain a sense of well-being, and establish connections within their community. Some of the key community resources and support services include:

1. Healthcare services: Access to healthcare services is critical for maintaining overall health and addressing ongoing medical needs. This may include primary care providers, specialist physicians, physical and occupational therapists, and mental health professionals. These services can help manage chronic conditions, monitor progress, and address any new health concerns that may arise during the reintegration process.
2. Support groups: Support groups provide a safe and supportive environment for individuals and their families to share their experiences, learn from one another, and build connections. These groups can be focused on specific conditions or challenges, such as brain injury, spinal cord injury, or stroke, or they may address broader topics, such as caregiver support or mental health. Participation in support groups can help individuals feel less isolated and better equipped to navigate their new circumstances.
3. Recreational programs: Adaptive recreational programs offer opportunities for individuals with disabilities or functional limitations to engage in physical, social, and leisure activities. These programs may include adaptive sports, art classes, music therapy, or other hobbies and interests. Participation in recreational programs can improve physical and mental well-being, enhance social connections, and promote overall quality of life.
4. Transportation services: Accessible transportation options are essential for community reintegration, as they enable individuals to attend medical appointments, access community resources, and participate in social and recreational activities. Rehabilitation

professionals can help patients and their families identify and navigate accessible transportation services in their community, such as paratransit programs or specialized transportation providers.
5. Financial assistance and benefits: Various financial assistance programs and benefits may be available to support individuals with disabilities and their families, such as Social Security Disability Insurance (SSDI), Supplemental Security Income (SSI), or other state and local assistance programs. Rehabilitation professionals can help patients and their families understand eligibility requirements and navigate the application process.
6. Educational and vocational services: For individuals looking to return to school or work, educational and vocational services can provide support in the form of accommodations, job training, and employment assistance. These services can help individuals achieve their educational and career goals, promoting independence and financial stability.

In conclusion, community resources and support services play a crucial role in facilitating successful community reintegration by addressing various aspects of a patient's life, from healthcare to social connections. Rehabilitation professionals can help patients and their families identify and access these resources, ensuring a smoother and more successful reintegration process.

Family education and support are essential components of the community reintegration process, as family members often play a significant role in providing care, assistance, and emotional support to individuals with disabilities or functional limitations. Ensuring that family members are well-informed and equipped to handle the challenges associated with community reintegration can greatly improve the overall success of the process and enhance the well-being of both the patient and their family. Key aspects of family education and support include:

1. Caregiver training: Family members who assume caregiving responsibilities may need training in various skills and techniques, such as safe transfer methods, medication administration, wound care, or adaptive equipment usage. Providing appropriate caregiver training can help family members feel more confident and competent in their caregiving role and reduce the risk of injury or complications.
2. Respite care: Caregiving can be physically, emotionally, and mentally demanding, and it is essential for caregivers to have access to regular breaks or periods of respite. Respite care services can offer temporary relief for caregivers, allowing them to rest, recharge, and attend to their personal needs. Respite care can be provided in various forms, such as in-home care, adult day programs, or short-term residential stays.
3. Emotional support: The emotional well-being of family members is just as important as that of the patient during the community reintegration process. Providing emotional support, such as counseling, support groups, or peer mentoring, can help family members process their feelings, cope with stress, and build resilience. Emotional support can also strengthen family relationships and promote a more positive home environment.

4. Family education: Family members should be educated about the patient's specific condition, functional limitations, and ongoing needs, as well as strategies for promoting independence and facilitating community reintegration. This education may be provided through individual consultations, group classes, or online resources. Family education can help to set realistic expectations, foster empathy, and promote a collaborative approach to problem-solving.
5. Navigating community resources: Rehabilitation professionals can help family members identify and access appropriate community resources and support services, such as healthcare providers, financial assistance programs, or recreational opportunities. By connecting families with these resources, professionals can help to alleviate some of the burden associated with community reintegration and ensure that families have the necessary support to navigate the process successfully.

In conclusion, family education and support play a crucial role in the community reintegration process by equipping family members with the knowledge, skills, and resources needed to effectively care for their loved ones and maintain their own well-being. By addressing the needs of both the patient and their family, rehabilitation professionals can help to promote successful community reintegration and enhance the overall quality of life for all involved.

Ongoing monitoring and follow-up are critical components of the community reintegration process, as they enable rehabilitation professionals, patients, and their families to evaluate progress, identify emerging challenges, and adapt care plans accordingly. Regular assessments and check-ins help ensure that individuals continue to receive the necessary support and resources to facilitate a successful reintegration. Key aspects of ongoing monitoring and follow-up include:

1. Assessing patient progress: It is essential to regularly assess the patient's progress in terms of functional abilities, emotional well-being, and social integration. This evaluation may involve the use of standardized assessment tools, observation, or self-report measures. By monitoring progress, rehabilitation professionals can identify areas where additional support or intervention may be needed.
2. Addressing emerging challenges: As individuals reintegrate into the community, new challenges may arise, such as changes in health status, evolving family dynamics, or unexpected barriers. Regular follow-up enables rehabilitation professionals to identify these challenges early and develop strategies to address them effectively, preventing setbacks or disruptions in the reintegration process.
3. Adjusting care plans: Based on the ongoing assessment of patient progress and emerging challenges, care plans may need to be adjusted or updated to better meet the individual's needs. This may involve modifying goals, implementing new interventions, or connecting the patient and family with additional community resources. Flexible and adaptive care planning helps to ensure that individuals receive the support they need to achieve optimal outcomes.
4. Maintaining interdisciplinary collaboration: Ongoing monitoring and follow-up provide opportunities for continued collaboration among the interdisciplinary team members

involved in the patient's care. Regular communication and information sharing among professionals help to facilitate a coordinated and integrated approach to care, enhancing the overall effectiveness of the reintegration process.
5. Supporting patient and family engagement: Regular follow-up also helps to maintain the engagement of the patient and their family in the reintegration process. It provides opportunities for them to ask questions, express concerns, and actively participate in decision-making, fostering a sense of empowerment and ownership over their care.

In summary, ongoing monitoring and follow-up are vital elements of the community reintegration process, as they enable rehabilitation professionals, patients, and their families to track progress, address challenges, and adapt care plans as needed. This proactive and responsive approach helps to ensure that individuals receive the support and resources necessary to achieve successful reintegration and improve their overall quality of life.

Promoting health equity and reducing disparities in community reintegration are crucial to ensuring that all individuals, regardless of their background or circumstances, have the opportunity to achieve optimal health outcomes. Culturally competent care and targeted interventions for underserved populations are essential components of this effort. Some strategies to promote health equity and reduce disparities in community reintegration include:

1. Culturally competent care: Health professionals should be sensitive to the cultural, social, and linguistic needs of diverse patient populations. This may involve providing care that is respectful of and responsive to patients' cultural beliefs, values, and communication preferences. Cultural competence training can help providers develop the necessary knowledge, skills, and attitudes to deliver culturally appropriate care.
2. Addressing social determinants of health: Social determinants of health, such as socioeconomic status, education, neighborhood environment, and access to healthcare, can have a significant impact on community reintegration outcomes. Health professionals should be aware of these factors and collaborate with community organizations to address them, such as by connecting patients with resources like affordable housing, transportation, and educational opportunities.
3. Targeted interventions for underserved populations: Tailoring interventions and support services to the unique needs of underserved populations, such as racial and ethnic minorities, individuals with low socioeconomic status, and people with disabilities, can help reduce disparities in community reintegration outcomes. This may involve developing culturally specific programs, using community health workers to engage with hard-to-reach populations, or providing additional resources for individuals facing multiple barriers to reintegration.
4. Inclusive policies and practices: Health organizations should adopt policies and practices that promote inclusivity and reduce disparities, such as by offering services in multiple languages, ensuring physical accessibility, and using patient-centered communication strategies that take into account diverse communication needs.
5. Community engagement and partnership: Building partnerships with community organizations, advocacy groups, and other stakeholders can help health professionals

better understand and address the unique needs of diverse populations. Engaging community members in the planning, implementation, and evaluation of reintegration programs can also help ensure that services are responsive to local needs and priorities.
6. Data collection and monitoring: Collecting and analyzing data on community reintegration outcomes by demographic factors, such as race, ethnicity, and socioeconomic status, can help identify disparities and inform targeted interventions. Regular monitoring and evaluation of programs and services can also help ensure that they are effective in reducing disparities and promoting health equity.

By implementing these strategies, health professionals can work toward promoting health equity and reducing disparities in community reintegration outcomes, ensuring that all individuals have the opportunity to achieve their full health potential.

In conclusion, community reintegration is a vital aspect of the rehabilitation process, enabling individuals to regain their independence and resume their roles within their families, workplaces, and communities. Rehabilitation nurses play a critical role in supporting patients and their families during this important transition by addressing a range of factors that influence successful reintegration.

Throughout this chapter, we have discussed the importance of identifying and addressing barriers to community reintegration, such as physical, cognitive, emotional, social, and environmental factors. We also highlighted the process of assessing a patient's readiness for community reintegration and developing a comprehensive, individualized reintegration plan that involves interdisciplinary collaboration and active patient and family involvement.

Moreover, we explored the essential roles of various healthcare professionals, such as physical and occupational therapists, in preparing patients for successful community reintegration. The significance of psychosocial support and counseling, vocational rehabilitation, and accessible housing and home modifications was also emphasized.

We delved into the various community resources and support services available to patients and their families, as well as the importance of family education and support. Ongoing monitoring and follow-up during community reintegration were identified as crucial components for assessing patient progress, addressing emerging challenges, and adjusting care plans as needed.

Lastly, we discussed strategies for promoting health equity and reducing disparities in community reintegration, including culturally competent care and targeted interventions for underserved populations. By understanding and addressing these key components, rehabilitation nurses can provide essential support to patients and their families, facilitating optimal outcomes and a successful transition back into the community.

Special Topics in Rehabilitation Nursing

In the field of rehabilitation nursing, there are numerous special topics that address the unique needs of various patient populations and clinical situations. These topics are essential for providing comprehensive, patient-centered care to diverse individuals, as they highlight specific challenges, care considerations, and evidence-based practices tailored to each situation. A thorough understanding of these special topics enables rehabilitation nurses to deliver effective and specialized care, ultimately promoting better patient outcomes and overall quality of life. Some of the special topics in rehabilitation nursing include:

- Traumatic brain injury
- Spinal cord injury
- Stroke
- Amputations
- Chronic pain
- Pediatric rehabilitation
- Geriatric rehabilitation
- Neurodegenerative disorders
- Psychiatric rehabilitation
- Cultural competence and health disparities
- Ethical and legal considerations
- Research and evidence-based practice
- Integration of technology in rehabilitation nursing

Each of these special topics addresses a specific area of rehabilitation nursing care, adding depth and nuance to the nurse's understanding of the patient's unique needs and challenges. By mastering these topics, rehabilitation nurses can enhance their clinical practice and improve the overall patient experience during the rehabilitation process. In the upcoming sections, we will delve deeper into these special topics, discussing their significance, care strategies, and the role of rehabilitation nursing in addressing the unique challenges faced by patients within each domain.

Rehabilitation nursing for patients with traumatic brain injuries (TBIs) requires specialized knowledge and skills to address the unique challenges and care considerations associated with this patient population. TBIs can range from mild concussions to severe injuries, with varying degrees of cognitive, emotional, and physical impairments.

Cognitive aspects: TBIs can result in cognitive deficits, such as memory loss, difficulty with attention and concentration, impaired problem-solving abilities, and decreased executive functioning. Rehabilitation nurses must be aware of these cognitive challenges and adapt their care and communication strategies accordingly. This may include simplifying instructions, using memory aids, and providing additional support and supervision during activities.

Emotional aspects: Patients with TBIs may experience emotional and psychological challenges, including mood swings, depression, anxiety, irritability, and changes in personality. Rehabilitation nurses play a crucial role in providing emotional support and helping patients develop coping strategies to manage these emotional challenges. They may also collaborate with mental health professionals and involve family members in the care process.

Physical aspects: Physical impairments resulting from TBIs can include motor deficits, balance issues, and sensory disturbances. Rehabilitation nurses work closely with physical and occupational therapists to develop and implement individualized care plans aimed at restoring physical functioning and promoting independence. They may also assist with mobility training, positioning, and equipment management.

In addition to addressing these specific aspects of care, rehabilitation nurses must also coordinate and collaborate with interdisciplinary teams, advocate for the patient's needs, and provide education and support to both patients and their families. By understanding and addressing the unique challenges faced by patients with TBIs, rehabilitation nurses can help facilitate recovery and improve overall quality of life.

Rehabilitation nursing for patients with spinal cord injuries (SCIs) involves addressing the specific needs and care strategies that focus on promoting mobility, independence, and quality of life. SCIs can result in varying degrees of paralysis and functional limitations, making it essential for rehabilitation nurses to be knowledgeable and skilled in handling the unique challenges associated with this patient population.

Mobility: Depending on the level and severity of the SCI, patients may experience partial or complete loss of mobility. Rehabilitation nurses play a pivotal role in helping patients regain as much movement as possible by collaborating with physical therapists, occupational therapists, and other healthcare professionals. They assist with mobility training, transfers, and the use of adaptive equipment, such as wheelchairs, braces, and assistive devices.

Independence: One of the primary goals of rehabilitation nursing for patients with SCIs is to help them achieve the highest level of independence possible. Nurses work with patients to develop self-care skills, such as bathing, dressing, and feeding, and they also help them learn to manage bowel and bladder function. Rehabilitation nurses provide education and support to patients and their families on using adaptive devices and making necessary modifications in their homes and daily routines.

Quality of life: Patients with SCIs often face significant challenges to their quality of life, including the potential for secondary complications such as pressure sores, urinary tract infections, and respiratory issues. Rehabilitation nurses are responsible for monitoring patients' overall health, managing symptoms, and implementing preventive measures to minimize the risk of complications. They also address psychosocial concerns, provide emotional support, and facilitate coping strategies to help patients and their families adjust to the life changes associated with an SCI.

In summary, rehabilitation nursing for patients with spinal cord injuries involves a comprehensive approach to care that addresses mobility, independence, and quality of life. By utilizing targeted care strategies and working closely with interdisciplinary teams, rehabilitation nurses can make a significant impact on the lives of patients with SCIs and support their journey toward recovery and adaptation.

Stroke rehabilitation nursing plays a crucial role in the care and recovery of stroke patients. Rehabilitation nurses address various aspects of care, including motor function, communication, and emotional support, to help patients regain their independence and achieve the best possible quality of life.

Motor function: Strokes often result in motor impairments, such as weakness or paralysis on one side of the body, difficulties with balance and coordination, and problems with fine motor skills. Rehabilitation nurses collaborate with physical and occupational therapists to design and implement individualized care plans aimed at improving patients' mobility, strength, and function. They also assist with exercises, transfers, and the use of adaptive equipment to promote safety and independence.

Communication: Stroke patients may experience communication difficulties, such as aphasia (language impairment) or dysarthria (speech impairment), which can be frustrating and isolating. Rehabilitation nurses work closely with speech and language therapists to support patients in regaining their communication abilities. Nurses play a vital role in facilitating communication by using alternative methods, such as communication boards or devices, and encouraging patients and their families to practice and develop new strategies.

Emotional support: The emotional impact of a stroke can be significant, with patients often experiencing feelings of depression, anxiety, and frustration. Rehabilitation nurses provide essential emotional support by listening to patients' concerns, validating their feelings, and offering encouragement throughout the recovery process. They may also collaborate with mental health professionals to ensure patients receive appropriate interventions for any psychological challenges they may face.

In addition to these specific aspects of care, stroke rehabilitation nursing involves coordinating with the interdisciplinary team, educating patients and their families about stroke prevention and self-management, and monitoring for potential complications. By addressing the unique needs of stroke patients and providing comprehensive, patient-centered care, rehabilitation nurses play a vital role in promoting recovery, fostering resilience, and enhancing overall well-being.

Rehabilitation nursing care for patients who have experienced **amputations** is a specialized area that focuses on addressing the unique challenges and needs of these individuals. Key aspects of this care include prosthetic fitting, mobility training, and psychological support, all of which contribute to promoting independence, self-confidence, and overall quality of life.

Prosthetic fitting: After an amputation, patients may be fitted with a prosthetic limb to help regain function and mobility. Rehabilitation nurses collaborate closely with prosthetists, physical therapists, and occupational therapists to ensure proper prosthetic fitting and alignment. They also provide education and guidance to patients and their families on prosthetic care, maintenance, and potential complications to monitor.

Mobility training: Regaining mobility and learning to navigate daily activities with a prosthetic limb are crucial aspects of rehabilitation for patients with amputations. Rehabilitation nurses support patients throughout this process, offering assistance with mobility exercises and collaborating with therapy teams to develop individualized plans that focus on strengthening, balance, and coordination. Nurses also help patients learn to use assistive devices and adapt to new ways of performing tasks, promoting independence and self-sufficiency.

Psychological support: The emotional and psychological impact of an amputation can be significant, with patients experiencing grief, depression, anxiety, and adjustment difficulties. Rehabilitation nurses provide essential emotional support by empathetically listening to patients' concerns, validating their feelings, and offering encouragement. They may also work with mental health professionals to ensure that patients receive appropriate counseling or therapeutic interventions to help them cope with the psychological challenges associated with their amputation.

In addition to these specific aspects of care, rehabilitation nursing for patients with amputations involves addressing other potential issues, such as pain management, wound care, and the prevention of complications. By providing comprehensive, patient-centered care that addresses the unique needs of individuals with amputations, rehabilitation nurses play a vital role in fostering resilience, promoting recovery, and improving overall well-being.

Rehabilitation nursing care for patients **with chronic pain** involves addressing the unique challenges these individuals face while promoting pain management, coping skills, and functional improvement. This holistic approach aims to enhance patients' overall well-being and quality of life.

Pain management: Effective pain management is essential in rehabilitation nursing for patients with chronic pain. Nurses work closely with patients, their families, and interdisciplinary teams to develop and implement individualized pain management plans. These plans may include pharmacological interventions, such as analgesics and anti-inflammatory medications, as well as non-pharmacological approaches like physical therapy, relaxation techniques, and complementary therapies (e.g., acupuncture, massage, or transcutaneous electrical nerve stimulation). Rehabilitation nurses monitor patients' responses to these interventions, adjusting treatment plans as needed to optimize pain relief and minimize side effects.

Coping skills: Chronic pain can significantly impact patients' emotional well-being, leading to feelings of frustration, depression, and anxiety. Rehabilitation nurses support patients in developing effective coping skills to manage the psychological aspects of chronic pain. This may involve providing education on stress management techniques, facilitating participation in support groups, or collaborating with mental health professionals to provide counseling and other therapeutic interventions. By fostering resilience and promoting healthy coping strategies, rehabilitation nurses help patients navigate the emotional challenges associated with chronic pain.

Functional improvement: Chronic pain can limit patients' ability to perform daily activities and maintain independence. Rehabilitation nurses focus on enhancing functional abilities by addressing limitations and promoting adaptive strategies. This may involve working with physical and occupational therapists to develop individualized exercise programs, mobility training, and techniques for energy conservation. Nurses also educate patients on strategies to prevent exacerbation of pain and promote self-management skills, empowering them to take an active role in their care.

In summary, rehabilitation nursing for patients with chronic pain encompasses a comprehensive, patient-centered approach that addresses pain management, coping skills, and functional improvement. By working closely with patients and interdisciplinary teams, rehabilitation nurses help individuals with chronic pain overcome challenges and improve their overall well-being and quality of life.

Pediatric rehabilitation nursing involves addressing the unique needs of children and adolescents during the rehabilitation process. This specialized field requires age-appropriate interventions, close family involvement, and a strong focus on developmental milestones to promote optimal recovery and well-being.

Age-appropriate interventions: Pediatric rehabilitation nurses must be knowledgeable about the specific physical, cognitive, and emotional needs of children at various stages of development. This understanding allows them to tailor interventions to the child's age, abilities, and interests. For example, therapeutic activities and exercises may be designed as games or playful tasks to engage younger children, while adolescents may respond better to goal-oriented tasks and autonomy in their rehabilitation plan.

Family involvement: The involvement of family members is crucial in pediatric rehabilitation nursing, as parents and caregivers play a significant role in supporting the child's recovery. Rehabilitation nurses work closely with families to educate them about the child's condition, treatment plan, and strategies for supporting the child at home. Family-centered care may also include addressing the emotional needs of parents and siblings, as the entire family may be affected by the child's illness or injury. By fostering a strong partnership between healthcare providers and families, pediatric rehabilitation nurses help create a supportive environment that facilitates the child's progress.

Developmental milestones: A key aspect of pediatric rehabilitation nursing is the assessment and promotion of developmental milestones. Children with illnesses or injuries may experience delays in reaching milestones, which can impact their overall growth and development. Rehabilitation nurses collaborate with interdisciplinary teams, including physical, occupational, and speech therapists, to design and implement interventions that target developmental milestones. These professionals monitor the child's progress and adjust the rehabilitation plan as needed to promote optimal development.

In summary, pediatric rehabilitation nursing focuses on the specific considerations and approaches necessary for addressing the unique needs of children and adolescents during the rehabilitation process. By incorporating age-appropriate interventions, engaging families, and targeting developmental milestones, pediatric rehabilitation nurses play a vital role in supporting the recovery and well-being of young patients.

Geriatric rehabilitation nursing focuses on the unique aspects of care for older adults during the rehabilitation process. It addresses age-related changes, comorbidities, and the promotion of independence and quality of life. Providing effective care to older adults requires a deep understanding of the specific challenges they face and the application of tailored strategies to support their needs.

Age-related changes: Older adults often experience a variety of age-related changes, such as decreased strength, reduced mobility, sensory impairments, and cognitive decline. Geriatric rehabilitation nurses must be knowledgeable about these changes and how they impact the rehabilitation process. By adapting interventions and strategies to accommodate age-related challenges, nurses can help older adults achieve the best possible outcomes.

Comorbidities: Many older adults have multiple chronic health conditions, which can complicate the rehabilitation process. Geriatric rehabilitation nurses must be skilled at managing comorbidities and addressing the interactions between different health conditions. This may involve coordinating care with various healthcare providers, adjusting medications, and monitoring for potential complications. By taking a holistic approach to care, nurses can help older adults manage their complex health needs while working towards rehabilitation goals.

Promotion of independence and quality of life: A key goal of geriatric rehabilitation nursing is to promote independence and enhance the quality of life for older adults. This involves identifying each individual's strengths and abilities, setting realistic goals, and developing a patient-centered care plan. Rehabilitation nurses may also work with older adults and their families to identify appropriate assistive devices, home modifications, and community resources that can support independence and participation in meaningful activities.

In summary, geriatric rehabilitation nursing focuses on the unique aspects of care for older adults during the rehabilitation process. By addressing age-related changes, managing comorbidities, and promoting independence and quality of life, geriatric rehabilitation nurses play a crucial role in supporting the well-being of older adults throughout their recovery journey.

Rehabilitation nursing for patients with **neurodegenerative** disorders involves a comprehensive approach to care that addresses the unique challenges faced by individuals living with conditions such as Parkinson's disease, multiple sclerosis, or other progressive neurological conditions. The focus is on symptom management, maximizing function, and improving the quality of life for patients and their families.

Symptom management: Neurodegenerative disorders often present with a wide range of symptoms that can vary in severity and progression. Rehabilitation nurses must be knowledgeable about these symptoms and work closely with other healthcare professionals to develop and implement individualized symptom management strategies. This may involve medication management, non-pharmacological interventions, and addressing secondary complications such as fatigue, pain, and mood disturbances.

Maximizing function: As neurodegenerative disorders progress, patients may experience a decline in their functional abilities. Rehabilitation nurses play a crucial role in helping patients maintain and improve their function through targeted interventions and adaptive strategies. This may include physical therapy to improve strength, balance, and mobility; occupational therapy to support activities of daily living and promote independence; and speech therapy to address communication and swallowing difficulties.

Supporting patients and families: Providing care for patients with neurodegenerative disorders can be challenging for families and caregivers, and rehabilitation nurses play an essential role in offering support and education. This may involve teaching families about the disease process, offering guidance on managing symptoms, and providing emotional support and counseling to help cope with the challenges of living with a progressive neurological condition.

Collaboration and coordination of care: Rehabilitation nursing for patients with neurodegenerative disorders often requires close collaboration with an interdisciplinary team of healthcare professionals, such as neurologists, therapists, and social workers. Rehabilitation nurses must be skilled in coordinating care, communicating with the team, and advocating for the needs of their patients to ensure a comprehensive and patient-centered approach to care.

In summary, rehabilitation nursing for patients with neurodegenerative disorders involves addressing the unique care considerations and strategies required for this patient population. By focusing on symptom management, maximizing function, supporting patients and families, and collaborating with an interdisciplinary team, rehabilitation nurses play a vital role in improving the lives of individuals living with these complex conditions.

Psychiatric rehabilitation nursing plays a crucial role in the care of patients with mental health conditions. Rehabilitation nurses work collaboratively with other healthcare professionals to help individuals achieve their highest level of functioning and well-being by addressing various aspects of recovery, including self-care, social skills, and community integration.

Self-care: Encouraging self-care is a significant aspect of psychiatric rehabilitation nursing. Nurses support patients in developing and maintaining daily routines, managing medications, and promoting healthy lifestyle habits, such as regular exercise, proper nutrition, and good sleep hygiene. By fostering self-care skills, rehabilitation nurses help patients regain a sense of control and autonomy over their lives.

Social skills: Effective social skills are essential for successful community living and overall well-being. Psychiatric rehabilitation nurses work with patients to develop and enhance social skills, such as effective communication, conflict resolution, and problem-solving. Group therapy sessions and social skills training programs can be beneficial in fostering interpersonal relationships and providing opportunities for patients to practice these skills in a supportive environment.

Community integration: One of the primary goals of psychiatric rehabilitation nursing is to help patients integrate successfully into their communities. This involves working closely with patients to identify meaningful activities, such as employment or volunteer opportunities, educational pursuits, and recreational activities. Nurses may also collaborate with community resources, such as housing programs, vocational rehabilitation services, and support groups, to assist patients in achieving their goals and building a supportive network.

Collaboration and coordination of care: Psychiatric rehabilitation nursing often requires close collaboration with an interdisciplinary team of healthcare professionals, including psychiatrists, psychologists, social workers, and occupational therapists. Rehabilitation nurses must effectively coordinate care, communicate with team members, and advocate for the needs of their patients to ensure a comprehensive and patient-centered approach to care.

Education and support for families: Families of individuals with mental health conditions can play a vital role in the recovery process. Psychiatric rehabilitation nurses provide education and support to families, helping them understand the nature of mental health conditions, the importance of treatment adherence, and strategies for coping with challenges related to caregiving.

In conclusion, psychiatric rehabilitation nursing is an essential component of care for patients with mental health conditions. By focusing on self-care, social skills, community integration, and working collaboratively with interdisciplinary teams, rehabilitation nurses contribute significantly to the recovery and well-being of individuals living with mental health conditions.

Integrating technology in rehabilitation nursing is transforming the way care is delivered, offering innovative solutions to enhance patient care and outcomes. Applications such as telehealth, assistive devices, and virtual reality are just a few examples of how technology is reshaping the field.

Telehealth: Telehealth has emerged as a valuable tool for rehabilitation nursing, enabling remote monitoring, consultations, and even therapy sessions. Telehealth can help bridge the gap for patients with limited access to specialized care, reduce the need for travel, and facilitate more frequent communication between healthcare providers and patients. This technology can also enable caregivers and family members to be more involved in the rehabilitation process, providing additional support and education.

Assistive devices: Technological advancements have led to the development of numerous assistive devices designed to improve function, independence, and quality of life for patients with various impairments. Examples include advanced prosthetics, powered exoskeletons, and adaptive equipment for self-care and mobility. Rehabilitation nurses play a key role in helping patients learn to use these devices effectively and incorporate them into their daily lives.

Virtual reality: Virtual reality (VR) technology is gaining traction in rehabilitation nursing, offering immersive and engaging environments for patients to practice functional skills, overcome fears, or relearn everyday tasks. VR can simulate real-life scenarios and provide immediate feedback, making it an effective tool for motor, cognitive, and emotional rehabilitation. By incorporating VR into the rehabilitation process, nurses can offer a novel approach to therapy that is both motivating and adaptable to each patient's unique needs.

Education and training: As technology continues to advance, it is essential for rehabilitation nurses to remain up-to-date on the latest tools and techniques available. Ongoing education and training will ensure that nurses are well-equipped to integrate technology into their practice, providing the best possible care for their patients.

In summary, technology is playing an increasingly important role in rehabilitation nursing, offering new and innovative ways to enhance patient care and outcomes. The integration of telehealth, assistive devices, and virtual reality has the potential to significantly impact the field, providing novel solutions for addressing patient needs and improving the overall rehabilitation experience.

Cultural competence and addressing health disparities are vital aspects of rehabilitation nursing, as they ensure that high-quality care is provided to diverse patient populations. Cultural competence refers to the ability of healthcare professionals to effectively interact with patients from different cultural backgrounds, while health disparities represent the differences in health outcomes and healthcare access experienced by various groups.

Importance of cultural competence in rehabilitation nursing:

1. Enhances patient-provider communication: Culturally competent rehabilitation nurses are better equipped to communicate with patients from different cultural backgrounds. This improved communication promotes trust, understanding, and ultimately better adherence to treatment plans.
2. Reduces misunderstandings and misinterpretations: A culturally competent rehabilitation nurse is aware of cultural beliefs and practices that could impact a patient's perception of illness, treatment, and recovery. By considering these factors, the nurse can tailor their approach and avoid misunderstandings that could hinder the rehabilitation process.
3. Improves patient satisfaction and outcomes: Culturally competent care has been shown to result in higher patient satisfaction and improved health outcomes. By understanding and respecting the cultural needs of patients, rehabilitation nurses can foster a more positive and effective therapeutic relationship.

Strategies for addressing health disparities in rehabilitation nursing:

1. Self-awareness and cultural sensitivity: Rehabilitation nurses should continuously reflect on their own cultural background and biases, working towards self-awareness and cultural sensitivity. This can help them develop a more empathetic approach to care that respects the diverse needs of their patients.
2. Education and training: Ongoing education and training in cultural competence are essential for rehabilitation nurses. This education should include understanding cultural differences, beliefs, and practices related to health and illness, as well as effective communication strategies for diverse patient populations.
3. Collaborative care: Rehabilitation nurses should collaborate with other healthcare professionals, including interpreters, cultural brokers, and community health workers, to better understand and address the unique needs of diverse patient populations. This collaborative approach can help bridge cultural gaps and promote equitable care.
4. Community outreach and engagement: Rehabilitation nurses can work with community organizations, advocacy groups, and other stakeholders to address health disparities and promote health equity. By engaging with the community, rehabilitation nurses can gain valuable insights into local needs and resources, as well as identify opportunities for collaboration and improvement.

In summary, cultural competence and addressing health disparities are essential components of rehabilitation nursing. By promoting culturally competent care and implementing strategies to reduce health disparities, rehabilitation nurses can ensure that all patients receive high-quality, equitable care that is tailored to their unique needs and preferences.

Ethical and legal considerations play a crucial role in rehabilitation nursing, as they guide nurses in making informed decisions, protecting patient rights, and maintaining professional boundaries. Here are some key ethical and legal issues that rehabilitation nurses may encounter in their practice:

1. Informed consent: Rehabilitation nurses must ensure that patients are provided with sufficient information to make informed decisions about their care. This involves explaining the benefits, risks, and alternatives of proposed interventions, and obtaining the patient's consent before proceeding.
2. Patient autonomy: Respecting patient autonomy means honoring their right to make decisions about their own care, even if the nurse disagrees with the choices. Rehabilitation nurses should support patients' preferences, while providing guidance and education to help them make informed decisions.
3. Confidentiality: Nurses are legally and ethically obligated to protect patient privacy and maintain confidentiality. This includes not disclosing personal or medical information without the patient's consent, except when required by law or to protect the patient or others from harm.
4. Ethical decision-making: Rehabilitation nurses may face ethical dilemmas when the best course of action is unclear or when different ethical principles conflict. In these situations, nurses should utilize ethical decision-making frameworks, consult with colleagues or ethics committees, and consider relevant laws and professional guidelines to arrive at an appropriate resolution.
5. Patient rights: Nurses must be aware of and uphold patient rights, such as the right to privacy, dignity, and respect. They should also advocate for patients when their rights are not being met, working to ensure that patients receive the care they deserve.
6. Professional boundaries: Rehabilitation nurses should establish and maintain professional boundaries with patients, avoiding relationships that could lead to conflicts of interest or compromise the therapeutic relationship. This includes being aware of power dynamics and avoiding actions that could be perceived as inappropriate or exploitative.
7. Documentation and reporting: Nurses are responsible for accurate and timely documentation of patient care, which is essential for legal and ethical reasons. They must also report any unethical or illegal
8. Ethical and legal considerations play a crucial role in rehabilitation nursing, as they guide nurses in making informed decisions, protecting patient rights, and maintaining professional boundaries. Here are some key ethical and legal issues that rehabilitation nurses may encounter in their practice:
9. Informed consent: Rehabilitation nurses must ensure that patients are provided with sufficient information to make informed decisions about their care. This involves explaining the benefits, risks, and alternatives of proposed interventions, and obtaining the patient's consent before proceeding.
10. Patient autonomy: Respecting patient autonomy means honoring their right to make decisions about their own care, even if the nurse disagrees with the choices.

Rehabilitation nurses should support patients' preferences, while providing guidance and education to help them make informed decisions.
11. Confidentiality: Nurses are legally and ethically obligated to protect patient privacy and maintain confidentiality. This includes not disclosing personal or medical information without the patient's consent, except when required by law or to protect the patient or others from harm.
12. Ethical decision-making: Rehabilitation nurses may face ethical dilemmas when the best course of action is unclear or when different ethical principles conflict. In these situations, nurses should utilize ethical decision-making frameworks, consult with colleagues or ethics committees, and consider relevant laws and professional guidelines to arrive at an appropriate resolution.
13. Patient rights: Nurses must be aware of and uphold patient rights, such as the right to privacy, dignity, and respect. They should also advocate for patients when their rights are not being met, working to ensure that patients receive the care they deserve.
14. Professional boundaries: Rehabilitation nurses should establish and maintain professional boundaries with patients, avoiding relationships that could lead to conflicts of interest or compromise the therapeutic relationship. This includes being aware of power dynamics and avoiding actions that could be perceived as inappropriate or exploitative.
15. Documentation and reporting: Nurses are responsible for accurate and timely documentation of patient care, which is essential for legal and ethical reasons. They must also report any unethical or illegal

Research and evidence-based practice play a crucial role in advancing the field of rehabilitation nursing, leading to the discovery of effective interventions, improved patient outcomes, and optimized care delivery. By integrating the latest research findings and best practices, rehabilitation nurses can ensure that their care is both clinically effective and patient-centered. The following are some key aspects of research and evidence-based practice in rehabilitation nursing:

1. Expanding knowledge base: Research contributes to the expansion of the knowledge base in rehabilitation nursing, leading to a deeper understanding of patient needs, interventions, and outcomes. It also helps identify gaps in current practice, guiding future research efforts.
2. Implementing evidence-based practice: Rehabilitation nurses are responsible for staying up-to-date with the latest research and integrating evidence-based practices into their care. This involves critically appraising research findings, synthesizing relevant evidence, and applying it to individual patient situations.
3. Quality improvement: Evidence-based practice plays a vital role in quality improvement initiatives, as it helps rehabilitation nurses identify areas for improvement, develop strategies for change, and evaluate the effectiveness of those changes.
4. Current trends: Some current trends in rehabilitation nursing research include the study of patient-centered care, telehealth, interdisciplinary collaboration, and the role of

technology in rehabilitation. These areas of research are shaping the future of rehabilitation nursing practice and may lead to new interventions and care models.
5. Future directions: Rehabilitation nursing research will continue to evolve, with an increasing focus on patient outcomes, personalized care, and the development of innovative interventions. Additionally, there may be greater emphasis on research that addresses health disparities, social determinants of health, and the needs of diverse patient populations.

By promoting research and evidence-based practice, rehabilitation nurses can contribute to the ongoing advancement of the field, ultimately enhancing patient care and outcomes.

This chapter highlighted the importance of understanding and addressing special topics in rehabilitation nursing to provide comprehensive, patient-centered care for diverse populations. Key points covered include:

1. Traumatic Brain Injury: Rehabilitation nurses must be aware of the unique challenges and care considerations for patients with traumatic brain injuries, addressing cognitive, emotional, and physical aspects of rehabilitation.
2. Spinal Cord Injury: Specific needs and care strategies for patients with spinal cord injuries must be addressed, focusing on mobility, independence, and quality of life.
3. Stroke Rehabilitation: Rehabilitation nursing plays a critical role in the care of stroke patients, including motor function, communication, and emotional support.
4. Amputations: Unique aspects of rehabilitation nursing care for patients with amputations involve prosthetic fitting, mobility training, and psychological support.
5. Chronic Pain: Rehabilitation nurses must address the challenges and strategies for providing care to patients with chronic pain, including pain management, coping skills, and functional improvement.
6. Pediatric and Geriatric Rehabilitation: Age-specific considerations and approaches in rehabilitation nursing for pediatric and geriatric patients are crucial, focusing on age-appropriate interventions, family involvement, and developmental milestones or age-related changes.
7. Neurodegenerative Disorders: Care considerations and strategies for patients with neurodegenerative disorders, such as Parkinson's disease and multiple sclerosis, involve symptom management and maximizing function.
8. Psychiatric Rehabilitation: Rehabilitation nursing plays a vital role in the care of patients with mental health conditions, emphasizing self-care, social skills, and community integration.
9. Technology Integration: Rehabilitation nursing is increasingly incorporating technology applications such as telehealth, assistive devices, and virtual reality to enhance patient care and outcomes.
10. Cultural Competence and Health Disparities: Cultural competence is vital in rehabilitation nursing, along with strategies for addressing health disparities among diverse patient populations.

11. Ethical and Legal Considerations: Rehabilitation nurses must be aware of and navigate ethical and legal issues that may arise in their practice.
12. Research and Evidence-Based Practice: Research and evidence-based practice are essential in advancing the field of rehabilitation nursing and ensuring optimal patient care.

By understanding these special topics, rehabilitation nurses can provide comprehensive, patient-centered care tailored to the unique needs of diverse populations, ultimately improving patient outcomes and quality of life.

Practice Exam Section:

Welcome to the practice exam section of this study guide! This section is designed to test your knowledge and understanding of the material covered throughout the guide, providing you with an opportunity to assess your readiness for the actual examination. The practice exam will consist of multiple-choice questions, carefully crafted to cover a wide range of topics from the chapters we've explored.

To enhance your learning experience and make this section as user-friendly as possible, we've decided to provide the correct answer and a brief explanation immediately following each question. This approach offers several benefits:

1. Immediate feedback: By providing the answer and explanation right after the question, you'll receive instant feedback on your response, allowing you to quickly identify areas where you may need further review or clarification.
2. Improved retention: Research has shown that immediate feedback can help enhance learning and memory retention. By understanding why an answer is correct or incorrect, you can better internalize the concepts and apply them in future situations.
3. Time efficiency: Having the answer and explanation readily available eliminates the need to flip back and forth between the questions and an answer key located at the end of the book. This saves you time and allows you to maintain your focus on the content.
4. Reduced frustration: Locating answers in a separate answer key can be frustrating, especially if you're unsure of the correct response. By providing the answer immediately after the question, we hope to minimize any frustration and keep you engaged in the learning process.

As you work through the practice exam, we encourage you to carefully read each question and the corresponding explanation, regardless of whether you answered correctly or not. This will help solidify your understanding of the material and better prepare you for success on the actual examination.

1. Which of the following best describes the primary purpose of models and theories in rehabilitation nursing practice?
a) To provide a rigid set of rules for nursing interventions
b) To predict patient outcomes with absolute certainty
c) To guide clinical decision-making and enhance patient outcomes
d) To replace the need for individualized patient assessments

Answer: c) To guide clinical decision-making and enhance patient outcomes

Explanation: Models and theories serve as a framework for rehabilitation nursing practice, helping to guide clinical decision-making and enhance patient outcomes. They do not provide rigid rules or predict outcomes with absolute certainty but rather offer a structured approach to understanding and addressing the unique needs of each patient.

2. How can rehabilitation nursing theories contribute to evidence-based practice?
a) By disregarding research findings in favor of anecdotal evidence
b) By providing a framework for organizing and interpreting research findings
c) By dictating a single, universally applicable intervention for all patients
d) By discouraging the use of clinical judgment in patient care

Answer: b) By providing a framework for organizing and interpreting research findings

Explanation: Rehabilitation nursing theories can contribute to evidence-based practice by providing a framework for organizing and interpreting research findings. This helps nurses integrate the latest research into their clinical practice, ensuring that they provide the most effective care for their patients.

3. Which of the following is NOT a characteristic of a useful rehabilitation nursing theory?
a) Applicable to a wide range of patient populations
b) Consistent with current research and evidence-based practice
c) Rigid and inflexible, with no room for adaptation
d) Considers the unique needs and goals of each patient

Answer: c) Rigid and inflexible, with no room for adaptation

Explanation: A useful rehabilitation nursing theory should be applicable to various patient populations, consistent with current research and evidence-based practice, and consider the unique needs and goals of each patient. It should not be rigid and inflexible, as this would limit its applicability and hinder the ability of nurses to provide individualized care.

4. Which aspect of rehabilitation nursing practice is most directly influenced by models and theories?
a) Billing and reimbursement processes
b) Interprofessional collaboration
c) Clinical decision-making
d) Facility design and layout

Answer: c) Clinical decision-making

Explanation: Models and theories most directly influence clinical decision-making in rehabilitation nursing practice. By providing a framework for understanding patient needs and guiding the selection of appropriate interventions, models and theories help nurses make informed decisions that promote optimal patient outcomes.

5. How can a strong understanding of rehabilitation nursing models and theories improve patient outcomes?
a) By eliminating the need for patient input in the care planning process
b) By ensuring that all patients receive the same standard set of interventions
c) By guiding the selection of appropriate, evidence-based interventions
d) By discouraging collaboration with other healthcare professionals

Answer: c) By guiding the selection of appropriate, evidence-based interventions

Explanation: A strong understanding of rehabilitation nursing models and theories can improve patient outcomes by guiding the selection of appropriate, evidence-based interventions. This allows nurses to provide individualized care that addresses each patient's unique needs and promotes their recovery and quality of life.

6. Which of the following best describes the concept of patient-centered care in rehabilitation nursing?
a) Making decisions for the patient without considering their preferences
b) Providing the same set of interventions for all patients, regardless of their individual needs
c) Prioritizing the needs and preferences of the patient in the planning and delivery of care
d) Limiting the involvement of the patient's family and support system in the care process

Answer: c) Prioritizing the needs and preferences of the patient in the planning and delivery of care

Explanation: Patient-centered care involves prioritizing the needs and preferences of the patient in the planning and delivery of care. It emphasizes the importance of involving the patient, their family, and support system in the decision-making process to ensure that care is tailored to their unique needs and goals.

7. Why is interdisciplinary collaboration important in rehabilitation nursing?
a) To reduce the workload for individual healthcare professionals
b) To ensure a comprehensive approach to patient care that addresses all aspects of a patient's needs
c) To create competition among healthcare professionals, which encourages better performance
d) To minimize the need for communication between healthcare professionals

Answer: b) To ensure a comprehensive approach to patient care that addresses all aspects of a patient's needs

Explanation: Interdisciplinary collaboration is important in rehabilitation nursing to ensure a comprehensive approach to patient care that addresses all aspects of a patient's needs. By working together, healthcare professionals from different disciplines can combine their expertise to develop and implement more effective care plans.

8. Which of the following is an example of a goal-oriented intervention in rehabilitation nursing?
a) Providing all patients with the same set of exercises, regardless of their individual abilities
b) Focusing on addressing a specific patient need or goal, such as improving mobility or self-care skills
c) Limiting the involvement of the patient in the goal-setting process
d) Ignoring the patient's progress and adjusting care plans only when absolutely necessary

Answer: b) Focusing on addressing a specific patient need or goal, such as improving mobility or self-care skills

Explanation: Goal-oriented interventions in rehabilitation nursing involve focusing on addressing specific patient needs or goals, such as improving mobility or self-care skills. This approach helps ensure that the care provided is tailored to the unique needs of each patient, promoting better outcomes and patient satisfaction.

9. How can a rehabilitation nurse best support the principle of patient-centered care?
a) By making all care decisions independently without consulting the patient or their support system
b) By involving the patient and their support system in the care planning process
c) By providing one-size-fits-all care, regardless of individual patient needs
d) By focusing solely on the medical aspects of care and ignoring the patient's psychosocial needs

Answer: b) By involving the patient and their support system in the care planning process

Explanation: A rehabilitation nurse can best support the principle of patient-centered care by involving the patient and their support system in the care planning process. This helps ensure that care is tailored to the unique needs and preferences of the patient, promoting better outcomes and patient satisfaction.

10. In the context of rehabilitation nursing, what is the primary purpose of goal-oriented interventions?
a) To provide a standardized approach to care for all patients
b) To focus on the achievement of specific patient outcomes and improvements
c) To minimize the need for ongoing care and support
d) To discourage collaboration among healthcare professionals

Answer: b) To focus on the achievement of specific patient outcomes and improvements

Explanation: The primary purpose of goal-oriented interventions in rehabilitation nursing is to focus on the achievement of specific patient outcomes and improvements. This approach helps ensure that care is tailored to the unique needs of each patient, promoting better outcomes and overall patient satisfaction.

11. What is the primary focus of Orem's Self-Care Deficit Theory in the context of rehabilitation nursing?
a) Encouraging patients to rely solely on nursing care for their needs
b) Identifying and addressing patients' self-care deficits to promote independence
c) Prioritizing the nurse's role in decision-making over the patient's preferences
d) Emphasizing the importance of the nurse's personal beliefs in providing care

Answer: b) Identifying and addressing patients' self-care deficits to promote independence.
Explanation: Orem's Self-Care Deficit Theory focuses on identifying and addressing patients' self-care deficits to promote independence. This theory is particularly relevant in rehabilitation nursing, as it emphasizes the importance of empowering patients to take an active role in their own care and recovery.

12. How does Roy's Adaptation Model relate to rehabilitation nursing practice?
a) It emphasizes the importance of nurses adapting their care to suit the needs of each patient
b) It focuses on helping patients adapt to changes in their health and environment as part of the rehabilitation process
c) It suggests that patients should adapt to the care provided by nurses, regardless of their preferences
d) It prioritizes the adaptation of nursing practices to align with the latest medical research

Answer: b) It focuses on helping patients adapt to changes in their health and environment as part of the rehabilitation process.
Explanation: Roy's Adaptation Model relates to rehabilitation nursing practice by focusing on helping patients adapt to changes in their health and environment as part of the rehabilitation process. This model emphasizes the importance of supporting patients in developing adaptive strategies to cope with new challenges and limitations.

13. Which of the following best describes Watson's Theory of Human Caring in the context of rehabilitation nursing?
a) It highlights the importance of providing care that is focused solely on physical health
b) It encourages nurses to disregard the emotional and psychological aspects of patient care
c) It emphasizes the need for nurses to develop caring relationships with patients and their families
d) It promotes the idea that nurses should prioritize their own well-being over that of their patients

Answer: c) It emphasizes the need for nurses to develop caring relationships with patients and their families

Explanation: Watson's Theory of Human Caring emphasizes the need for nurses to develop caring relationships with patients and their families in the context of rehabilitation nursing. This theory highlights the importance of addressing not only the physical aspects of patient care but also the emotional and psychological aspects, which are integral to the healing process.

14. How does Orem's Self-Care Deficit Theory differ from Watson's Theory of Human Caring in the context of rehabilitation nursing?
a) Orem's theory focuses on self-care deficits, while Watson's theory emphasizes caring relationships
b) Orem's theory highlights the importance of the nurse's beliefs, while Watson's theory focuses on patient preferences
c) Orem's theory emphasizes physical health, while Watson's theory focuses on emotional and psychological aspects of care
d) Orem's theory prioritizes medical research, while Watson's theory emphasizes the need for personal adaptation

Answer: a) Orem's theory focuses on self-care deficits, while Watson's theory emphasizes caring relationships

Explanation: Orem's Self-Care Deficit Theory differs from Watson's Theory of Human Caring in that Orem's theory focuses on identifying and addressing patients' self-care deficits to promote independence, while Watson's theory emphasizes the need for nurses to develop caring relationships with patients and their families, addressing emotional and psychological aspects of care.

15. How can rehabilitation nurses apply the principles of Roy's Adaptation Model in their practice?
a) By expecting patients to adapt to the care provided without considering their individual needs
b) By focusing solely on the medical aspects of care and ignoring patients' psychological needs
c) By helping patients develop adaptive strategies to cope with changes in their health and environment
d) By prioritizing the development of new nursing theories over implementing existing models

Answer: c) By helping patients develop adaptive strategies to cope with changes in their health and environment
Explanation: Rehabilitation nurses can apply the principles of Roy's Adaptation Model in their practice by helping patients develop adaptive strategies to cope with changes in their health and environment. This involves supporting patients in adjusting to new challenges and limitations as part of the rehabilitation process, as well as collaborating with interdisciplinary team members to create individualized care plans that address the unique needs of each patient.

16. The Biopsychosocial Model is used in rehabilitation nursing to:
a) Focus solely on the physical aspects of a patient's condition
b) Emphasize the psychological and social aspects of a patient's condition over their physical well-being
c) Consider the complex interactions between a patient's biological, psychological, and social factors
d) Replace all other nursing theories and models

Answer: c) Consider the complex interactions between a patient's biological, psychological, and social factors

Explanation: The Biopsychosocial Model takes into account the complex interactions between a patient's biological, psychological, and social factors. By considering all these aspects, rehabilitation nurses can develop comprehensive care plans that address the patient's physical, emotional, and social needs.

17. The Disablement Model in rehabilitation nursing primarily focuses on:
a) Minimizing the impact of disabilities on a patient's life
b) Identifying the root causes of disabilities
c) Encouraging patients to ignore their disabilities
d) Focusing solely on the medical treatment of disabilities

Answer: a) Minimizing the impact of disabilities on a patient's life

Explanation: The Disablement Model aims to minimize the impact of disabilities on a patient's life by focusing on the functional limitations and restrictions they face. Rehabilitation nurses use this model to guide their interventions, helping patients adapt and overcome the challenges associated with their disabilities.

18. The International Classification of Functioning, Disability, and Health (ICF) is used in rehabilitation nursing to:
a) Classify different types of nursing theories
b) Provide a standardized framework for understanding and measuring health and disability
c) Offer a comprehensive list of nursing interventions
d) Act as a diagnostic tool for identifying disabilities

Answer: b) Provide a standardized framework for understanding and measuring health and disability

Explanation: The ICF provides a standardized framework for understanding and measuring health and disability. It is used in rehabilitation nursing to assess patients' functioning, identify their needs and goals, and guide the development of individualized care plans that promote optimal outcomes.

19. One key benefit of using the Biopsychosocial Model in rehabilitation nursing is:
a) It ignores the patient's social and psychological well-being
b) It simplifies the rehabilitation process by focusing only on physical aspects
c) It helps identify the patient's support system and resources
d) It replaces the need for interdisciplinary collaboration

Answer: c) It helps identify the patient's support system and resources

Explanation: By considering the complex interactions between a patient's biological, psychological, and social factors, the Biopsychosocial Model helps rehabilitation nurses identify the patient's support system and resources, which can be crucial in developing a comprehensive and effective care plan.

20. Which of the following is a key principle of the Disablement Model in rehabilitation nursing?
a) Emphasizing the patient's medical diagnosis over functional limitations
b) Encouraging patients to focus on their disabilities
c) Identifying and addressing the functional limitations and restrictions related to a patient's disability
d) Ignoring the impact of disabilities on a patient's daily life

Answer: c) Identifying and addressing the functional limitations and restrictions related to a patient's disability

Explanation: The Disablement Model focuses on identifying and addressing the functional limitations and restrictions related to a patient's disability. This approach allows rehabilitation nurses to develop tailored interventions that help patients overcome the challenges associated with their disabilities and improve their overall quality of life.

21. In an acute care setting, the primary focus of rehabilitation nursing is to:
a) Provide long-term, comprehensive care for patients with chronic conditions
b) Facilitate a smooth transition to a subacute care facility or outpatient setting
c) Address the immediate medical needs of patients with life-threatening conditions
d) Oversee the day-to-day management of patients' disabilities in a home setting

Answer: b) Facilitate a smooth transition to a subacute care facility or outpatient setting

Explanation: In an acute care setting, rehabilitation nursing focuses on stabilizing the patient's condition and facilitating a smooth transition to a subacute care facility or outpatient setting, where they will receive ongoing rehabilitation services tailored to their individual needs and goals.

22. The primary goal of rehabilitation nursing in subacute care is to:
a) Provide intensive, short-term rehabilitation services
b) Address long-term disability management needs
c) Focus solely on patients' medical diagnoses
d) Facilitate an immediate return to the patient's prior level of functioning

Answer: a) Provide intensive, short-term rehabilitation services
Explanation: In a subacute care setting, rehabilitation nursing primarily focuses on providing intensive, short-term rehabilitation services aimed at helping patients regain their functional abilities and maximize their independence before transitioning to a less intensive care setting or returning home.

23. Rehabilitation nursing in outpatient clinics typically involves:
a) Providing round-the-clock nursing care
b) Developing and implementing long-term disability management plans
c) Offering specialized, goal-oriented rehabilitation services on an outpatient basis
d) Coordinating care exclusively within a hospital setting

Answer: c) Offering specialized, goal-oriented rehabilitation services on an outpatient basis
Explanation: In outpatient clinics, rehabilitation nursing focuses on offering specialized, goal-oriented rehabilitation services on an outpatient basis. This allows patients to receive the necessary interventions while maintaining their regular routines and living in their own homes.

24. Home care rehabilitation nursing primarily aims to:
a) Manage acute medical emergencies in a home setting
b) Provide continuous supervision and care for patients with complex medical needs
c) Support patients in maintaining their independence and quality of life in their own homes
d) Offer intensive, short-term rehabilitation services

Answer: c) Support patients in maintaining their independence and quality of life in their own homes
Explanation: Home care rehabilitation nursing aims to support patients in maintaining their independence and quality of life in their own homes. Rehabilitation nurses assess patients' needs, develop individualized care plans, and provide necessary interventions to help patients adapt to their environment and manage their disabilities.

25. The application of rehabilitation nursing theories and models across different practice settings is important because:
a) It ensures a consistent approach to patient care
b) It eliminates the need for interdisciplinary collaboration
c) It allows for a one-size-fits-all approach to rehabilitation
d) It focuses solely on the medical aspects of care

Answer: a) It ensures a consistent approach to patient care

Explanation: Applying rehabilitation nursing theories and models across different practice settings ensures a consistent approach to patient care. This consistency helps rehabilitation nurses provide comprehensive, patient-centered care that addresses the unique needs and goals of each individual, regardless of the setting in which they receive care.

26. Rehabilitation nursing models and theories promote interdisciplinary collaboration by:
a) Encouraging a hierarchical approach to patient care
b) Focusing solely on nursing interventions and goals
c) Emphasizing the unique contributions of each team member in achieving patient goals
d) Discouraging communication between healthcare professionals

Answer: c) Emphasizing the unique contributions of each team member in achieving patient goals

Explanation: Rehabilitation nursing models and theories promote interdisciplinary collaboration by emphasizing the unique contributions of each team member in achieving patient goals. This approach fosters open communication, mutual respect, and collaboration among healthcare professionals.

27. An important aspect of interdisciplinary collaboration in rehabilitation nursing is:
a) Sharing patient information only when necessary
b) Developing individualized care plans without input from other team members
c) Participating in regular interdisciplinary team meetings
d) Assuming that all team members have the same understanding of the patient's needs

Answer: c) Participating in regular interdisciplinary team meetings

Explanation: Regular interdisciplinary team meetings are essential for effective collaboration in rehabilitation nursing. These meetings provide an opportunity for healthcare professionals to share information, discuss patient progress, and adjust care plans as needed to ensure optimal patient outcomes.

28. A rehabilitation nurse collaborates with a physical therapist to:
a) Manage a patient's medications
b) Develop and implement a mobility training plan
c) Address the patient's emotional and psychosocial needs
d) Assess the patient's nutritional status

Answer: b) Develop and implement a mobility training plan

Explanation: Rehabilitation nurses collaborate with physical therapists to develop and implement mobility training plans for patients. This collaboration ensures that interventions are tailored to the patient's unique needs and goals, promoting functional improvement and independence.

29. In collaborating with an occupational therapist, a rehabilitation nurse might focus on:
a) Developing strategies for managing chronic pain
b) Assessing and addressing cognitive deficits
c) Facilitating the patient's return to work or school
d) Coordinating the patient's discharge planning process

Answer: c) Facilitating the patient's return to work or school

Explanation: Rehabilitation nurses collaborate with occupational therapists to help patients return to work or school by identifying barriers, developing strategies to overcome them, and providing necessary support to ensure a successful transition.

30. When working with a social worker, a rehabilitation nurse may:
a) Perform a thorough physical assessment of the patient
b) Develop a comprehensive exercise program for the patient
c) Address financial, housing, and other social needs of the patient
d) Prescribe medications for symptom management

Answer: c) Address financial, housing, and other social needs of the patient

Explanation: Rehabilitation nurses collaborate with social workers to address financial, housing, and other social needs of patients. This collaboration helps to ensure that patients have access to the resources and support necessary for optimal recovery and quality of life.

31. Rehabilitation nursing theories play a crucial role in patient assessment by:
a) Providing a standardized approach for all patients
b) Focusing solely on the patient's physical needs
c) Encouraging a holistic view of the patient, considering biopsychosocial factors
d) Limiting the scope of the assessment to nursing interventions

Answer: c) Encouraging a holistic view of the patient, considering biopsychosocial factors
Explanation: Rehabilitation nursing theories encourage a holistic view of the patient, considering biopsychosocial factors. This approach helps nurses to identify and address the complex and interrelated needs of patients with disabilities or chronic conditions, leading to more effective care plans and interventions.

32. When setting goals for a patient's rehabilitation, a nurse guided by rehabilitation nursing theories would most likely:
a) Set goals based solely on the patient's medical diagnosis
b) Focus on goals related only to physical function
c) Develop goals without considering the patient's preferences or values
d) Establish patient-centered goals that address various aspects of the patient's life

Answer: d) Establish patient-centered goals that address various aspects of the patient's life
Explanation: Rehabilitation nursing theories emphasize patient-centered goal-setting, which involves considering the patient's preferences, values, and various aspects of their life. This approach leads to more meaningful and achievable goals that promote optimal patient outcomes.

33. When developing an individualized care plan for a patient, a rehabilitation nurse guided by rehabilitation nursing theories would:
a) Create a plan based on their personal experience and intuition
b) Focus exclusively on short-term goals and interventions
c) Consider only the patient's physical needs and limitations
d) Collaborate with the patient and interdisciplinary team to develop a comprehensive plan

Answer: d) Collaborate with the patient and interdisciplinary team to develop a comprehensive plan
Explanation: Rehabilitation nursing theories guide nurses to collaborate with the patient and interdisciplinary team in developing a comprehensive, individualized care plan. This approach ensures that the plan addresses the patient's unique needs and goals, promoting optimal outcomes.

34. According to rehabilitation nursing theories, an important aspect of patient assessment is:
a) Relying solely on objective data gathered from medical records
b) Ignoring the patient's psychosocial and emotional well-being
c) Gathering information about the patient's strengths and resources, as well as challenges
d) Focusing only on the patient's deficits and limitations

Answer: c) Gathering information about the patient's strengths and resources, as well as challenges
Explanation: Rehabilitation nursing theories emphasize the importance of gathering information about the patient's strengths and resources, as well as challenges, during the assessment process. This comprehensive approach helps nurses to identify opportunities for intervention and support that can enhance the patient's overall well-being and recovery.

35. When using rehabilitation nursing theories to guide goal setting, it is important to:
a) Set vague, general goals that can apply to any patient
b) Establish goals that are measurable, realistic, and time-bound
c) Focus on goals that are primarily determined by the healthcare team
d) Set goals that address only the patient's most immediate needs

Answer: b) Establish goals that are measurable, realistic, and time-bound

Explanation: Rehabilitation nursing theories emphasize the importance of setting goals that are measurable, realistic, and time-bound. This approach helps to ensure that goals are achievable, relevant, and focused on the patient's specific needs and priorities, leading to more effective interventions and better patient outcomes.

36. Rehabilitation nursing theories contribute to evidence-based practice by:
a) Encouraging nurses to rely on personal experience rather than research evidence
b) Providing a framework for evaluating and applying research findings
c) Discouraging the use of new interventions until they are well-established
d) Focusing solely on traditional nursing interventions

Answer: b) Providing a framework for evaluating and applying research findings

Explanation: Rehabilitation nursing theories provide a framework for evaluating and applying research findings, thus contributing to evidence-based practice. This ensures that nursing interventions are grounded in the best available evidence, leading to more effective patient care and improved outcomes.

37. When using evidence-based practice in rehabilitation nursing, a nurse should:
a) Rely solely on personal experience and clinical judgment
b) Ignore research findings that contradict their pre-existing beliefs
c) Apply research evidence selectively, based on their individual preferences
d) Continuously update their practice based on the best available evidence

Answer: d) Continuously update their practice based on the best available evidence

Explanation: Evidence-based practice in rehabilitation nursing involves continuously updating one's practice based on the best available evidence. This approach ensures that nursing interventions are informed by the latest research findings and best practices, resulting in improved patient care and outcomes.

38. In the context of rehabilitation nursing theories and evidence-based practice, a key benefit of using research evidence to inform nursing interventions is:
a) Reducing the need for interdisciplinary collaboration
b) Ensuring that interventions are more effective and relevant to the patient's needs
c) Eliminating the need for critical thinking and decision-making in nursing practice
d) Minimizing the importance of patient preferences and values

Answer: b) Ensuring that interventions are more effective and relevant to the patient's needs

Explanation: Using research evidence to inform nursing interventions, guided by rehabilitation nursing theories, ensures that interventions are more effective and relevant to the patient's needs. This approach enhances patient care and promotes better outcomes by grounding nursing practice in the best available evidence.

39. The relationship between rehabilitation nursing theories and evidence-based practice can be described as:
a) Antagonistic, with theories undermining the importance of research evidence
b) Complementary, with theories providing a foundation for applying research evidence
c) Unrelated, with theories and evidence-based practice addressing separate aspects of nursing
d) Competitive, with theories and evidence-based practice offering alternative approaches to nursing care

Answer: b) Complementary, with theories providing a foundation for applying research evidence
Explanation: Rehabilitation nursing theories and evidence-based practice have a complementary relationship. Theories provide a foundation for evaluating and applying research evidence, helping to ensure that nursing interventions are grounded in the best available evidence and promoting improved patient care and outcomes.

40. To enhance the integration of evidence-based practice in rehabilitation nursing, it is important to:
a) Focus exclusively on quantitative research findings
b) Prioritize personal experience over research evidence
c) Encourage critical appraisal and application of research findings
d) Rely on a single, universally accepted rehabilitation nursing theory

Answer: c) Encourage critical appraisal and application of research findings
Explanation: To enhance the integration of evidence-based practice in rehabilitation nursing, it is important to encourage critical appraisal and application of research findings. This approach promotes the use of the best available evidence to inform nursing interventions and supports continuous improvement in patient care and outcomes.

41. A rehabilitation nurse is using Orem's Self-Care Deficit Theory to guide the care of a patient recovering from a stroke. The nurse identifies that the patient is unable to perform self-care activities due to weakness in the affected limbs. Based on Orem's theory, the nurse should prioritize which intervention?
a) Implementing a complete dependence care plan
b) Encouraging the patient to perform self-care tasks independently
c) Providing partial assistance while gradually increasing patient responsibility
d) Focusing solely on improving the patient's physical abilities

Answer: c) Providing partial assistance while gradually increasing patient responsibility

Explanation: Orem's Self-Care Deficit Theory emphasizes the importance of patient-centered care, aiming to help patients regain their ability to perform self-care tasks. In this case, the nurse should prioritize providing partial assistance while gradually increasing patient responsibility, promoting self-care, and fostering independence.

42. A patient with a spinal cord injury is being cared for by a rehabilitation nurse who is using the Biopsychosocial Model to guide their practice. Which of the following interventions aligns with this model?
a) Focusing solely on physical therapy to improve the patient's mobility
b) Addressing only the psychological impact of the injury on the patient
c) Collaborating with the interdisciplinary team to address the patient's physical, psychological, and social needs
d) Disregarding the patient's cultural background and personal beliefs

Answer: c) Collaborating with the interdisciplinary team to address the patient's physical, psychological, and social needs

Explanation: The Biopsychosocial Model emphasizes the interconnectedness of physical, psychological, and social factors in patient care. A rehabilitation nurse using this model would collaborate with the interdisciplinary team to address the patient's comprehensive needs, including physical, psychological, and social aspects of care.

43. A rehabilitation nurse is applying the International Classification of Functioning, Disability, and Health (ICF) model to the care of a patient with multiple sclerosis. Which of the following interventions aligns with the ICF model?
a) Focusing exclusively on treating the patient's symptoms
b) Ignoring the patient's environmental and personal factors
c) Considering the patient's functioning, disability, and health in the context of their environment and personal factors
d) Disregarding the patient's goals and preferences for care

Answer: c) Considering the patient's functioning, disability, and health in the context of their environment and personal factors

Explanation: The ICF model takes a comprehensive approach to patient care, considering the patient's functioning, disability, and health in the context of their environment and personal factors. A rehabilitation nurse applying this model would consider all these aspects when planning and implementing care for a patient with multiple sclerosis.

44. A patient with a traumatic brain injury is receiving care from a rehabilitation nurse who uses Watson's Theory of Human Caring to guide their practice. Which of the following actions by the nurse aligns with this theory?
a) Focusing solely on the patient's physical needs and medical treatment
b) Establishing a caring, therapeutic relationship with the patient and their family
c) Ignoring the patient's emotional needs and focusing only on their cognitive abilities
d) Neglecting the importance of self-care and personal well-being for the nurse

Answer: b) Establishing a caring, therapeutic relationship with the patient and their family

Explanation: Watson's Theory of Human Caring emphasizes the importance of establishing a caring, therapeutic relationship with the patient and their family. A rehabilitation nurse using this theory would prioritize building a supportive, empathetic, and compassionate relationship with the patient and their family to promote healing and well-being.

45. provide a comprehensive framework for assessing and addressing patients' needs. Which of the following best describes the primary purpose of functional health patterns in rehabilitation nursing?
a) To focus exclusively on patients' physical health and well-being
b) To identify and address only patients' psychological needs
c) To provide a holistic approach to patient assessment and care planning
d) To disregard the impact of patients' social and environmental factors

Answer: c) To provide a holistic approach to patient assessment and care planning

Explanation: Functional health patterns allow rehabilitation nurses to take a holistic approach to patient assessment and care planning, considering various aspects of a patient's life, including physical, psychological, and social factors.

46. Which of the following is NOT considered a functional health pattern in rehabilitation nursing?
a) Nutrition and metabolism
b) Sleep and rest
c) Role and relationships
d) Medication administration

Answer: d) Medication administration

Explanation: Medication administration is an essential aspect of patient care, but it does not constitute a functional health pattern. Functional health patterns focus on broader aspects of a patient's well-being, such as nutrition, sleep, and relationships.

47. When conducting an assessment using functional health patterns, a rehabilitation nurse should prioritize:
a) Only the patient's physical health and functioning
b) The patient's psychological state, ignoring their physical needs
c) A single aspect of the patient's life, such as their social relationships
d) A comprehensive and holistic understanding of the patient's needs and strengths

Answer: d) A comprehensive and holistic understanding of the patient's needs and strengths

Explanation: Functional health patterns are designed to provide a comprehensive and holistic understanding of the patient's needs and strengths, taking into account various aspects of their life and well-being.

48. Which functional health pattern focuses on a patient's ability to express and manage emotions effectively?
a) Cognitive-perceptual
b) Coping and stress tolerance
c) Self-perception and self-concept
d) Activity and exercise

Answer: b) Coping and stress tolerance

Explanation: The coping and stress tolerance functional health pattern focuses on a patient's ability to express and manage emotions effectively, including their ability to cope with stress and adapt to change.

49. A rehabilitation nurse is using functional health patterns to assess a patient who has recently undergone surgery for a hip replacement. Which functional health pattern would be most relevant for addressing the patient's mobility and ability to perform daily activities?
a) Activity and exercise
b) Nutrition and metabolism
c) Sleep and rest
d) Role and relationships

Answer: a) Activity and exercise

Explanation: The activity and exercise functional health pattern focuses on a patient's mobility, physical activity, and ability to perform daily activities. This would be the most relevant pattern for addressing the needs of a patient recovering from hip replacement surgery.

50. A rehabilitation nurse is working with a patient who has recently had a stroke. The nurse decides to use the Biopsychosocial Model to guide their assessment and interventions. Which of the following elements will the nurse consider when using this model?
a) Only the patient's physical functioning
b) Only the patient's emotional and psychological state
c) The patient's physical functioning and their social environment, but not their emotional state
d) The patient's physical functioning, emotional and psychological state, and their social environment

Answer: d) The patient's physical functioning, emotional and psychological state, and their social environment

Explanation: The Biopsychosocial Model takes a comprehensive approach to patient care, considering the patient's physical functioning, emotional and psychological state, and their social environment as interrelated components that influence their overall well-being and recovery.

51. A rehabilitation nurse is planning care for a patient who has recently been diagnosed with a spinal cord injury. Which nursing theory would be most appropriate to guide the nurse in promoting the patient's self-care and independence?
a) Orem's Self-Care Deficit Theory
b) Roy's Adaptation Model
c) Watson's Theory of Human Caring
d) The Disablement Model

Answer: a) Orem's Self-Care Deficit Theory

Explanation: Orem's Self-Care Deficit Theory focuses on promoting self-care and independence in patients by identifying and addressing their self-care deficits. This theory would be most appropriate for guiding the nurse in planning care for a patient with a spinal cord injury who requires support in developing self-care skills.

52. A rehabilitation nurse is working with an interdisciplinary team to develop a care plan for a patient with a traumatic brain injury. The International Classification of Functioning, Disability, and Health (ICF) model is being used to guide the team's approach. What is the primary focus of the ICF model?
a) Identifying and addressing only the patient's physical impairments
b) Focusing on the patient's psychological state and ignoring their physical needs
c) Emphasizing the patient's disability rather than their abilities and strengths
d) Considering the patient's functioning within the context of their environment and personal factors

Answer: d) Considering the patient's functioning within the context of their environment and personal factors

Explanation: The ICF model focuses on understanding the patient's functioning within the context of their environment and personal factors, taking a holistic approach to patient care that considers various aspects of the patient's life and well-being.

53. The Disablement Model is being used by a rehabilitation nurse to guide the assessment and intervention for a patient with chronic pain. Which of the following best describes the focus of the Disablement Model?
a) Identifying and addressing the underlying cause of the patient's pain
b) Exploring the patient's personal and environmental factors that contribute to their pain experience
c) Focusing solely on the patient's psychological response to their pain
d) Ignoring the impact of the patient's pain on their daily functioning

Answer: b) Exploring the patient's personal and environmental factors that contribute to their pain experience. Explanation: The Disablement Model focuses on understanding the impact of a patient's condition on their daily functioning, considering personal and environmental factors that may contribute to their experience of pain and disability.

54. Which of the following best describes the purpose of functional health patterns in rehabilitation nursing?
a) To focus solely on the patient's physical needs
b) To address only the patient's emotional and psychological needs
c) To provide a structured framework for assessing and addressing patients' needs across multiple dimensions
d) To disregard the patient's social environment

Answer: c) To provide a structured framework for assessing and addressing patients' needs across multiple dimensions
Explanation: Functional health patterns provide a comprehensive and structured framework for assessing and addressing the diverse needs of patients in rehabilitation nursing, considering multiple dimensions such as physical, emotional, and social factors.

55. A rehabilitation nurse is using functional health patterns to assess a patient's nutritional and metabolic patterns. Which aspect of the patient's care is the nurse primarily concerned with in this context?
a) The patient's sleep and rest patterns
b) The patient's ability to perform activities of daily living
c) The patient's dietary intake, hydration, and metabolic needs
d) The patient's relationships and social support

Answer: c) The patient's dietary intake, hydration, and metabolic needs

Explanation: When assessing a patient's nutritional and metabolic patterns, the rehabilitation nurse focuses on aspects related to dietary intake, hydration, and metabolic needs, ensuring that the patient's nutritional status supports their overall health and recovery.

56. Which functional health pattern is primarily concerned with a patient's ability to express and manage their emotions?
a) Health perception-health management pattern
b) Sleep-rest pattern
c) Coping-stress tolerance pattern
d) Cognitive-perceptual pattern

Answer: c) Coping-stress tolerance pattern

Explanation: The coping-stress tolerance pattern focuses on a patient's ability to express and manage their emotions, as well as their capacity to cope with stressors related to their health condition and rehabilitation process.

57. A rehabilitation nurse is using functional health patterns to assess a patient's role-relationship pattern. Which of the following aspects would the nurse likely consider in this assessment?
a) The patient's perception of their self-concept and body image
b) The patient's ability to communicate effectively with others
c) The patient's social roles, relationships, and support systems
d) The patient's mobility and ability to perform activities of daily living

Answer: c) The patient's social roles, relationships, and support systems

Explanation: In the assessment of a patient's role-relationship pattern, the nurse focuses on the patient's social roles, relationships, and support systems, evaluating how these factors may influence the patient's rehabilitation process and overall well-being.

58. How do functional health patterns contribute to the development of individualized care plans in rehabilitation nursing?
a) By ignoring the patient's unique needs and preferences
b) By focusing only on the patient's physical functioning
c) By providing a comprehensive and multidimensional approach to patient assessment
d) By prioritizing the patient's psychological needs over their physical needs

Answer: c) By providing a comprehensive and multidimensional approach to patient assessment

Explanation: Functional health patterns support the development of individualized care plans by offering a comprehensive and multidimensional approach to patient assessment, allowing the rehabilitation nurse to identify and address the diverse needs of patients across various dimensions of their lives.

59. Marjory Gordon's Functional Health Patterns framework is comprised of how many distinct patterns?
a) 5
b) 8
c) 11
d) 15

Answer: c) 11
Explanation: Marjory Gordon's Functional Health Patterns framework consists of 11 distinct patterns, which provide a comprehensive approach to patient assessment and care planning in rehabilitation nursing practice.

60. Which of the following best describes the primary goal of using Gordon's Functional Health Patterns in rehabilitation nursing practice?
a) To diagnose medical conditions
b) To provide a standardized approach to patient assessment and care planning
c) To focus on the patient's physical needs only
d) To prioritize the patient's social needs over their physical needs

Answer: b) To provide a standardized approach to patient assessment and care planning
Explanation: The primary goal of using Gordon's Functional Health Patterns in rehabilitation nursing practice is to provide a standardized, comprehensive approach to patient assessment and care planning that addresses the diverse needs of patients across various dimensions.

61. In the context of Gordon's Functional Health Patterns, which pattern focuses on a patient's perception of their health status and their ability to manage their own health?
a) Sleep-rest pattern
b) Health perception-health management pattern
c) Cognitive-perceptual pattern
d) Role-relationship pattern

Answer: b) Health perception-health management pattern. Explanation: The health perception-health management pattern focuses on the patient's perception of their health status and their ability to manage their own health, including their understanding of their condition, adherence to treatment plans, and engagement in health-promoting behaviors.

62. A rehabilitation nurse using Gordon's Functional Health Patterns identifies issues related to a patient's ability to communicate effectively with others. Which functional health pattern is most relevant to this concern?
a) Self-perception-self-concept pattern
b) Value-belief pattern
c) Communication pattern
d) Activity-exercise pattern

Answer: c) Communication pattern. Explanation: The communication pattern within Gordon's Functional Health Patterns focuses on a patient's ability to communicate effectively with others, including verbal and non-verbal communication, as well as potential barriers to effective communication.

63. How does the use of Gordon's Functional Health Patterns contribute to the development of patient-centered care plans in rehabilitation nursing?
a) By focusing only on the patient's physical needs
b) By ignoring the patient's unique needs and preferences
c) By providing a comprehensive and individualized approach to patient assessment
d) By prioritizing the patient's psychological needs over their physical needs

Answer: c) By providing a comprehensive and individualized approach to patient assessment. Explanation: The use of Gordon's Functional Health Patterns in rehabilitation nursing contributes to the development of patient-centered care plans by providing a comprehensive and individualized approach to patient assessment, which enables the nurse to identify and address the diverse needs of patients across various dimensions of their lives.

64. Which of the following best describes the Health Perception-Health Management Pattern in Gordon's Functional Health Patterns?
a) The patient's ability to perform daily activities and exercise
b) The patient's perception of their health and ability to manage their care
c) The patient's quality and quantity of sleep and rest
d) The patient's coping mechanisms and stress management strategies

Answer: b) The patient's perception of their health and ability to manage their care
Explanation: The Health Perception-Health Management Pattern in Gordon's Functional Health Patterns focuses on the patient's perception of their health status and their ability to manage their care, including understanding their condition, adherence to treatment plans, and engagement in health-promoting behaviors.

65. How does assessing the Health Perception-Health Management Pattern contribute to a patient's rehabilitation?
a) By identifying potential barriers to successful rehabilitation outcomes
b) By providing a complete understanding of the patient's cognitive abilities
c) By prioritizing the patient's physical needs over their psychological needs
d) By focusing on the patient's relationships and social support systems

Answer: a) By identifying potential barriers to successful rehabilitation outcomes

Explanation: Assessing the Health Perception-Health Management Pattern contributes to a patient's rehabilitation by identifying potential barriers to successful outcomes, such as lack of understanding of their condition, non-adherence to treatment plans, or limited engagement in health-promoting behaviors.

66. Which of the following factors is most relevant to the Health Perception-Health Management Pattern in rehabilitation nursing?
a) The patient's level of mobility and independence
b) The patient's adherence to prescribed medications and treatments
c) The patient's ability to communicate effectively with others
d) The patient's values and beliefs about health and illness

Answer: b) The patient's adherence to prescribed medications and treatments

Explanation: The Health Perception-Health Management Pattern is most concerned with factors related to the patient's understanding of their health status and their ability to manage their care, including adherence to prescribed medications and treatments.

67. A rehabilitation nurse identifies that a patient has poor understanding of their health status and struggles to manage their care. What would be an appropriate intervention based on the Health Perception-Health Management Pattern?
a) Encourage the patient to engage in regular exercise
b) Provide education and resources to improve the patient's understanding of their condition
c) Address any sleep disturbances the patient may be experiencing
d) Facilitate communication between the patient and their healthcare team

Answer: b) Provide education and resources to improve the patient's understanding of their condition

Explanation: An appropriate intervention based on the Health Perception-Health Management Pattern would be to provide education and resources to improve the patient's understanding of their condition and ability to manage their care, which can ultimately contribute to better rehabilitation outcomes.

68. In the context of the Health Perception-Health Management Pattern, what is the primary goal of rehabilitation nursing interventions?
a) To improve the patient's physical functioning and independence
b) To enhance the patient's understanding of their health status and ability to manage their care
c) To support the patient's coping mechanisms and stress management strategies
d) To foster effective communication between the patient and their healthcare team

Answer: b) To enhance the patient's understanding of their health status and ability to manage their care

Explanation: The primary goal of rehabilitation nursing interventions in the context of the Health Perception-Health Management Pattern is to enhance the patient's understanding of their health status and ability to manage their care, which can contribute to better rehabilitation outcomes and overall well-being.

69. The Nutritional-Metabolic Pattern in Gordon's Functional Health Patterns is primarily concerned with which of the following aspects of patient care?
a) The patient's ability to manage their health and adhere to treatment plans
b) The patient's nutritional status and metabolic needs
c) The patient's ability to communicate effectively with their healthcare team
d) The patient's ability to perform daily activities and exercise

Answer: b) The patient's nutritional status and metabolic needs

Explanation: The Nutritional-Metabolic Pattern in Gordon's Functional Health Patterns focuses on assessing a patient's nutritional status and metabolic needs, which can play a critical role in their overall health and rehabilitation outcomes.

70. Which of the following is a key component of assessing the Nutritional-Metabolic Pattern in rehabilitation nursing?
a) Evaluating the patient's level of pain and discomfort
b) Identifying any difficulties the patient may have with swallowing or chewing
c) Assessing the patient's cognitive abilities and problem-solving skills
d) Examining the patient's social support systems and coping mechanisms

Answer: b) Identifying any difficulties the patient may have with swallowing or chewing

Explanation: Assessing the Nutritional-Metabolic Pattern in rehabilitation nursing includes identifying any difficulties the patient may have with swallowing or chewing, which can affect their ability to maintain adequate nutrition and may require intervention.

71. How does addressing the Nutritional-Metabolic Pattern contribute to successful rehabilitation outcomes?
a) By enhancing the patient's understanding of their health status and ability to manage their care
b) By promoting proper nutrition, which supports the healing process and overall well-being
c) By fostering effective communication between the patient and their healthcare team
d) By improving the patient's physical functioning and independence

Answer: b) By promoting proper nutrition, which supports the healing process and overall well-being

Explanation: Addressing the Nutritional-Metabolic Pattern contributes to successful rehabilitation outcomes by promoting proper nutrition, which supports the healing process, overall well-being, and functional improvement.

72. A patient in a rehabilitation setting has a poor appetite and is not meeting their nutritional needs. Which of the following interventions is most appropriate based on the Nutritional-Metabolic Pattern?
a) Encourage the patient to participate in group therapy sessions
b) Collaborate with a dietitian to develop a tailored meal plan to address the patient's preferences and nutritional needs
c) Provide education on the importance of exercise and physical activity
d) Offer resources to help the patient manage stress and cope with their health condition

Answer: b) Collaborate with a dietitian to develop a tailored meal plan to address the patient's preferences and nutritional needs

Explanation: Based on the Nutritional-Metabolic Pattern, an appropriate intervention for a patient with a poor appetite would be to collaborate with a dietitian to develop a tailored meal plan that addresses the patient's preferences and nutritional needs, supporting their overall health and rehabilitation progress.

73. In the context of the Nutritional-Metabolic Pattern, which of the following factors is most relevant when evaluating a patient's metabolic needs?
a) The patient's weight and body composition
b) The patient's level of social interaction and support
c) The patient's ability to adhere to prescribed medications and treatments
d) The patient's cognitive functioning and memory

Answer: a) The patient's weight and body composition

Explanation: When evaluating a patient's metabolic needs in the context of the Nutritional-Metabolic Pattern, the patient's weight and body composition are most relevant, as they can influence the individual's energy needs, nutritional requirements, and overall health.

74. Which of the following best describes the focus of the Elimination Pattern in rehabilitation nursing?
a) Assessing a patient's cognitive and emotional status
b) Evaluating a patient's nutritional intake and metabolism
c) Examining a patient's bowel, bladder, and skin function
d) Analyzing a patient's social support systems and coping mechanisms

Answer: c) Examining a patient's bowel, bladder, and skin function

Explanation: The Elimination Pattern in rehabilitation nursing focuses on assessing a patient's bowel, bladder, and skin function, which are essential aspects of a patient's overall health and well-being.

75. A patient in a rehabilitation setting is experiencing urinary incontinence. This issue is most directly related to which of Gordon's Functional Health Patterns?
a) Health Perception-Health Management Pattern
b) Nutritional-Metabolic Pattern
c) Elimination Pattern
d) Activity-Exercise Pattern

Answer: c) Elimination Pattern

Explanation: Urinary incontinence is most directly related to the Elimination Pattern, as it involves the assessment and management of bladder function in rehabilitation nursing.

76. In the context of the Elimination Pattern, which of the following interventions is most appropriate for a patient with constipation?
a) Encourage increased fluid intake and physical activity
b) Provide education on stress management techniques
c) Assess the patient's social support and coping mechanisms
d) Evaluate the patient's cognitive abilities and memory

Answer: a) Encourage increased fluid intake and physical activity

Explanation: In the context of the Elimination Pattern, encouraging increased fluid intake and physical activity can help alleviate constipation by promoting regular bowel movements.

77. Which of the following factors is most relevant when assessing a patient's skin function as part of the Elimination Pattern?
a) The patient's level of pain and discomfort
b) The patient's ability to manage their own healthcare needs
c) The presence of pressure ulcers or skin breakdown
d) The patient's dietary preferences and eating habits

Answer: c) The presence of pressure ulcers or skin breakdown
Explanation: Assessing a patient's skin function as part of the Elimination Pattern includes evaluating the presence of pressure ulcers or skin breakdown, as these issues can negatively impact the patient's overall health and rehabilitation progress.

78. How does addressing the Elimination Pattern contribute to successful rehabilitation outcomes?
a) By promoting effective communication between the patient and their healthcare team
b) By ensuring that the patient's nutritional needs are met
c) By preventing complications and promoting comfort related to bowel, bladder, and skin function
d) By enhancing the patient's understanding of their health status and ability to manage their care

Answer: c) By preventing complications and promoting comfort related to bowel, bladder, and skin function
Explanation: Addressing the Elimination Pattern contributes to successful rehabilitation outcomes by preventing complications and promoting comfort related to bowel, bladder, and skin function, which can impact a patient's overall well-being and ability to participate in rehabilitation activities.

79. The Activity-Exercise Pattern in rehabilitation nursing primarily focuses on assessing:
a) A patient's cognitive abilities and memory
b) A patient's social support systems and coping mechanisms
c) A patient's functional abilities, mobility, and exercise tolerance
d) A patient's nutritional status and metabolic needs

Answer: c) A patient's functional abilities, mobility, and exercise tolerance
Explanation: The Activity-Exercise Pattern in rehabilitation nursing primarily focuses on assessing a patient's functional abilities, mobility, and exercise tolerance, which are critical factors in determining a patient's rehabilitation potential and progress.

80. Which of the following is an essential component of evaluating a patient's Activity-Exercise Pattern in the context of rehabilitation nursing?
a) Assessing the patient's ability to perform activities of daily living (ADLs)
b) Evaluating the patient's understanding of their health status
c) Determining the patient's dietary preferences and eating habits
d) Identifying the patient's sources of social support

Answer: a) Assessing the patient's ability to perform activities of daily living (ADLs)

Explanation: Assessing a patient's ability to perform activities of daily living (ADLs) is an essential component of evaluating their Activity-Exercise Pattern, as it provides insight into their functional abilities and independence in daily tasks.

81. A patient in a rehabilitation setting has limited mobility and requires assistance with transfers. This issue is most directly related to which of Gordon's Functional Health Patterns?
a) Health Perception-Health Management Pattern
b) Nutritional-Metabolic Pattern
c) Elimination Pattern
d) Activity-Exercise Pattern

Answer: d) Activity-Exercise Pattern

Explanation: Limited mobility and requiring assistance with transfers are most directly related to the Activity-Exercise Pattern, as they involve assessing and managing a patient's mobility and functional abilities in rehabilitation nursing.

82. In the context of the Activity-Exercise Pattern, which of the following interventions is most appropriate for a patient with decreased exercise tolerance?
a) Encourage increased fluid intake and physical activity
b) Provide education on stress management techniques
c) Assess the patient's social support and coping mechanisms
d) Develop a graded exercise program to improve endurance

Answer: d) Develop a graded exercise program to improve endurance

Explanation: In the context of the Activity-Exercise Pattern, developing a graded exercise program to improve endurance is an appropriate intervention for a patient with decreased exercise tolerance, as it can help enhance their ability to participate in rehabilitation activities.

83. How does addressing the Activity-Exercise Pattern contribute to successful rehabilitation outcomes?
a) By promoting effective communication between the patient and their healthcare team
b) By ensuring that the patient's nutritional needs are met
c) By preventing complications related to bowel, bladder, and skin function
d) By maximizing a patient's functional abilities, mobility, and participation in rehabilitation activities

Answer: d) By maximizing a patient's functional abilities, mobility, and participation in rehabilitation activities

Explanation: Addressing the Activity-Exercise Pattern contributes to successful rehabilitation outcomes by maximizing a patient's functional abilities, mobility, and participation in rehabilitation activities, which are essential for achieving independence and improving quality of life.

84. In the context of rehabilitation nursing, addressing the Sleep-Rest Pattern is essential because:
a) It helps identify the patient's dietary preferences and eating habits
b) It promotes effective communication between the patient and healthcare team
c) It aids in optimizing the patient's energy levels and ability to participate in rehabilitation activities
d) It helps prevent complications related to bowel, bladder, and skin function

Answer: c) It aids in optimizing the patient's energy levels and ability to participate in rehabilitation activities

Explanation: Addressing the Sleep-Rest Pattern in rehabilitation nursing is essential because it can help optimize the patient's energy levels and ability to participate in rehabilitation activities, thus improving their overall rehabilitation experience and outcomes.

85. A rehabilitation nurse is assessing a patient's Sleep-Rest Pattern. Which of the following factors should be considered?
a) The patient's ability to perform activities of daily living (ADLs)
b) The patient's frequency and consistency of bowel movements
c) The patient's sleep quality, rest habits, and overall energy levels
d) The patient's understanding of their health status

Answer: c) The patient's sleep quality, rest habits, and overall energy levels

Explanation: When assessing a patient's Sleep-Rest Pattern, the rehabilitation nurse should consider factors such as the patient's sleep quality, rest habits, and overall energy levels, as these are directly related to the Sleep-Rest Pattern and can impact their participation in rehabilitation activities.

86. Which of the following interventions is most appropriate for addressing sleep disturbances in a rehabilitation setting?
a) Encourage increased fluid intake and physical activity
b) Implement a consistent sleep schedule and promote sleep hygiene
c) Assess the patient's social support and coping mechanisms
d) Develop a graded exercise program to improve endurance

Answer: b) Implement a consistent sleep schedule and promote sleep hygiene

Explanation: Implementing a consistent sleep schedule and promoting sleep hygiene is an appropriate intervention for addressing sleep disturbances in a rehabilitation setting, as it can help improve sleep quality and support the patient's overall energy levels.

87. A patient in a rehabilitation setting is experiencing excessive daytime sleepiness. This issue is most directly related to which of Gordon's Functional Health Patterns?
a) Health Perception-Health Management Pattern
b) Nutritional-Metabolic Pattern
c) Elimination Pattern
d) Sleep-Rest Pattern

Answer: d) Sleep-Rest Pattern

Explanation: Excessive daytime sleepiness is most directly related to the Sleep-Rest Pattern, as it involves assessing and managing a patient's sleep quality, rest habits, and overall energy levels in rehabilitation nursing.

88. How does optimizing the Sleep-Rest Pattern contribute to successful rehabilitation outcomes?
a) By promoting effective communication between the patient and their healthcare team
b) By ensuring that the patient's nutritional needs are met
c) By preventing complications related to bowel, bladder, and skin function
d) By enhancing the patient's energy levels, which supports participation in rehabilitation activities

Answer: d) By enhancing the patient's energy levels, which supports participation in rehabilitation activities

Explanation: Optimizing the Sleep-Rest Pattern contributes to successful rehabilitation outcomes by enhancing the patient's energy levels, which supports their ability to participate in rehabilitation activities and, in turn, improves their overall rehabilitation experience and outcomes.

89. The primary focus of the Cognitive-Perceptual Pattern in rehabilitation nursing is to:
a) Assess and address a patient's nutritional needs
b) Evaluate and support a patient's cognitive abilities, sensory-perceptual function, and communication skills
c) Determine a patient's ability to manage their own care
d) Optimize a patient's sleep quality and energy levels

Answer: b) Evaluate and support a patient's cognitive abilities, sensory-perceptual function, and communication skills

Explanation: The Cognitive-Perceptual Pattern in rehabilitation nursing is primarily focused on evaluating and supporting a patient's cognitive abilities, sensory-perceptual function, and communication skills, as these factors can greatly impact the patient's rehabilitation process and overall quality of life.

90. Which of the following assessments is most relevant to the Cognitive-Perceptual Pattern in rehabilitation nursing?
a) Assessing a patient's level of mobility and exercise tolerance
b) Evaluating a patient's ability to swallow and chew food
c) Determining a patient's bowel and bladder function
d) Administering cognitive and sensory-perceptual screening tests

Answer: d) Administering cognitive and sensory-perceptual screening tests

Explanation: Administering cognitive and sensory-perceptual screening tests is the most relevant assessment for the Cognitive-Perceptual Pattern in rehabilitation nursing, as these tests help to identify any cognitive or sensory-perceptual deficits that may impact the patient's ability to engage in rehabilitation activities and achieve their goals.

91. A rehabilitation nurse is working with a patient who has difficulty communicating due to aphasia. This challenge is directly related to which of Gordon's Functional Health Patterns?
a) Health Perception-Health Management Pattern
b) Nutritional-Metabolic Pattern
c) Elimination Pattern
d) Cognitive-Perceptual Pattern

Answer: d) Cognitive-Perceptual Pattern

Explanation: Difficulty communicating due to aphasia is directly related to the Cognitive-Perceptual Pattern, as this pattern addresses a patient's cognitive abilities, sensory-perceptual function, and communication skills in rehabilitation nursing.

92. In the context of rehabilitation nursing, an appropriate intervention for a patient with visual impairment would be:
a) Providing alternative communication strategies and devices
b) Implementing environmental modifications to improve safety and navigation
c) Encouraging a consistent sleep schedule and sleep hygiene
d) Developing a graded exercise program to improve endurance

Answer: b) Implementing environmental modifications to improve safety and navigation

Explanation: Implementing environmental modifications to improve safety and navigation is an appropriate intervention for a patient with visual impairment in the context of rehabilitation nursing, as it addresses the sensory-perceptual aspect of the Cognitive-Perceptual Pattern, ensuring that the patient can safely engage in rehabilitation activities.

93. A rehabilitation nurse identifies that a patient has difficulty with memory and attention. To address this issue, the nurse should implement interventions related to which Functional Health Pattern?
a) Health Perception-Health Management Pattern
b) Nutritional-Metabolic Pattern
c) Elimination Pattern
d) Cognitive-Perceptual Pattern

Answer: d) Cognitive-Perceptual Pattern

Explanation: If a patient has difficulty with memory and attention, the rehabilitation nurse should implement interventions related to the Cognitive-Perceptual Pattern, as this pattern focuses on evaluating and supporting a patient's cognitive abilities, sensory-perceptual function, and communication skills in rehabilitation nursing.

94. The Self-Perception-Self-Concept Pattern is primarily concerned with assessing and addressing a patient's:
a) Cognitive abilities and sensory-perceptual function
b) Self-image, self-esteem, and emotional well-being
c) Nutritional status and metabolic needs
d) Mobility, functional abilities, and exercise tolerance

Answer: b) Self-image, self-esteem, and emotional well-being

Explanation: The Self-Perception-Self-Concept Pattern focuses on understanding a patient's self-image, self-esteem, and emotional well-being in the rehabilitation setting, as these factors can significantly impact the patient's engagement in the rehabilitation process and overall recovery.

95. Which of the following interventions is most relevant to the Self-Perception-Self-Concept Pattern in rehabilitation nursing?
a) Facilitating a support group for patients with similar disabilities or conditions
b) Developing an individualized exercise program
c) Assessing and monitoring a patient's bowel and bladder function
d) Administering cognitive and sensory-perceptual screening tests

Answer: a) Facilitating a support group for patients with similar disabilities or conditions

Explanation: Facilitating a support group for patients with similar disabilities or conditions is an intervention that directly addresses the Self-Perception-Self-Concept Pattern, as it helps patients to share experiences, build self-esteem, and improve their emotional well-being.

96. A patient in a rehabilitation setting expresses feelings of low self-worth due to their disability. This concern is related to which of Gordon's Functional Health Patterns?
a) Health Perception-Health Management Pattern
b) Nutritional-Metabolic Pattern
c) Self-Perception-Self-Concept Pattern
d) Sleep-Rest Pattern

Answer: c) Self-Perception-Self-Concept Pattern

Explanation: A patient's feelings of low self-worth due to their disability are related to the Self-Perception-Self-Concept Pattern, which focuses on understanding and addressing a patient's self-image, self-esteem, and emotional well-being in the rehabilitation setting.

97. A rehabilitation nurse identifies that a patient is experiencing depression and feelings of isolation due to their disability. To address this issue, the nurse should implement interventions related to which Functional Health Pattern?
a) Health Perception-Health Management Pattern
b) Nutritional-Metabolic Pattern
c) Self-Perception-Self-Concept Pattern
d) Sleep-Rest Pattern

Answer: c) Self-Perception-Self-Concept Pattern

Explanation: If a patient is experiencing depression and feelings of isolation due to their disability, the rehabilitation nurse should implement interventions related to the Self-Perception-Self-Concept Pattern, which focuses on understanding and addressing a patient's self-image, self-esteem, and emotional well-being in the rehabilitation setting.

98. Which of the following assessments is most relevant to the Self-Perception-Self-Concept Pattern in rehabilitation nursing?
a) Administering a standardized self-esteem questionnaire
b) Assessing a patient's mobility and exercise tolerance
c) Evaluating a patient's nutritional status and metabolic needs
d) Determining a patient's sleep quality and rest habits

Answer: a) Administering a standardized self-esteem questionnaire

Explanation: Administering a standardized self-esteem questionnaire is the most relevant assessment for the Self-Perception-Self-Concept Pattern in rehabilitation nursing, as it helps to identify any self-image, self-esteem, or emotional well-being issues that may impact the patient's engagement in the rehabilitation process and overall recovery.

99. The Roles-Relationships Pattern in rehabilitation nursing is primarily focused on assessing and addressing a patient's:
a) Social functioning and support systems
b) Sleep quality and rest habits
c) Cognitive abilities and sensory-perceptual function
d) Nutritional status and metabolic needs

Answer: a) Social functioning and support systems

Explanation: The Roles-Relationships Pattern is centered on evaluating a patient's social functioning, support systems, and ability to maintain or adapt to their roles in the context of rehabilitation nursing.

100. A rehabilitation nurse identifies that a patient is struggling to adapt to their new role as a person with a disability. Which of Gordon's Functional Health Patterns is most relevant to addressing this issue?
a) Health Perception-Health Management Pattern
b) Nutritional-Metabolic Pattern
c) Roles-Relationships Pattern
d) Sleep-Rest Pattern

Answer: c) Roles-Relationships Pattern

Explanation: The Roles-Relationships Pattern is most relevant to addressing a patient's struggle to adapt to their new role as a person with a disability, as it focuses on social functioning, support systems, and the ability to maintain or adapt to roles in the context of rehabilitation nursing.

101. Which of the following interventions is most appropriate for a rehabilitation nurse to implement when addressing the Roles-Relationships Pattern?
a) Encouraging the patient to participate in group therapy sessions
b) Developing a personalized exercise program
c) Assessing the patient's bowel and bladder function
d) Administering cognitive and sensory-perceptual screening tests

Answer: a) Encouraging the patient to participate in group therapy sessions

Explanation: Encouraging the patient to participate in group therapy sessions is an appropriate intervention for addressing the Roles-Relationships Pattern, as it provides opportunities for social interaction, support, and the development of coping strategies related to their roles and relationships.

102. A patient in a rehabilitation setting is having difficulty maintaining their pre-injury relationships due to changes in their physical abilities. This concern is related to which of Gordon's Functional Health Patterns?
a) Health Perception-Health Management Pattern
b) Nutritional-Metabolic Pattern
c) Roles-Relationships Pattern
d) Sleep-Rest Pattern

Answer: c) Roles-Relationships Pattern

Explanation: A patient's difficulty maintaining pre-injury relationships due to changes in their physical abilities is related to the Roles-Relationships Pattern, which focuses on evaluating and addressing a patient's social functioning, support systems, and ability to maintain or adapt to their roles in the context of rehabilitation nursing.

103. Which assessment tool is most relevant to the Roles-Relationships Pattern in rehabilitation nursing?
a) A standardized social support questionnaire
b) A mobility and exercise tolerance test
c) A nutritional status and metabolic needs assessment
d) A sleep quality and rest habits survey

Answer: a) A standardized social support questionnaire

Explanation: A standardized social support questionnaire is the most relevant assessment tool for the Roles-Relationships Pattern in rehabilitation nursing, as it helps to identify the patient's social functioning, support systems, and ability to maintain or adapt to their roles in the context of rehabilitation nursing.

104. The primary focus of the Sexuality-Reproductive Pattern in rehabilitation nursing is to assess and address a patient's:
a) Social functioning and support systems
b) Nutritional status and metabolic needs
c) Sexual health and reproductive function
d) Sleep quality and rest habits

Answer: c) Sexual health and reproductive function

Explanation: The Sexuality-Reproductive Pattern primarily focuses on evaluating and addressing a patient's sexual health and reproductive function in the context of rehabilitation nursing.

105. A patient with a spinal cord injury is concerned about their ability to maintain sexual relationships post-injury. Which of Gordon's Functional Health Patterns is most relevant to addressing this issue?
a) Health Perception-Health Management Pattern
b) Nutritional-Metabolic Pattern
c) Roles-Relationships Pattern
d) Sexuality-Reproductive Pattern

Answer: d) Sexuality-Reproductive Pattern

Explanation: The Sexuality-Reproductive Pattern is most relevant to addressing a patient's concerns about their ability to maintain sexual relationships post-injury, as it focuses on assessing and addressing sexual health and reproductive function in rehabilitation nursing.

106. In addressing the Sexuality-Reproductive Pattern, a rehabilitation nurse might:
a) Encourage the patient to join a support group for individuals with similar injuries
b) Develop a personalized exercise program
c) Provide education on adaptive sexual techniques and devices
d) Administer cognitive and sensory-perceptual screening tests
Answer: c) Provide education on adaptive sexual techniques and devices

Explanation: Providing education on adaptive sexual techniques and devices is a suitable intervention for addressing the Sexuality-Reproductive Pattern, as it helps patients overcome barriers and maintain sexual health and reproductive function in the context of rehabilitation nursing.

107. Which assessment tool is most relevant to the Sexuality-Reproductive Pattern in rehabilitation nursing?
a) A standardized social support questionnaire
b) A mobility and exercise tolerance test
c) A nutritional status and metabolic needs assessment
d) A sexual health and function questionnaire

Answer: d) A sexual health and function questionnaire

Explanation: A sexual health and function questionnaire is the most relevant assessment tool for the Sexuality-Reproductive Pattern in rehabilitation nursing, as it helps to identify the patient's sexual health and reproductive function in the context of rehabilitation nursing.

108. The primary goal of assessing the Coping-Stress Tolerance Pattern in rehabilitation nursing is to understand a patient's:
a) Sleep quality and rest habits
b) Social functioning and support systems
c) Coping strategies, stress tolerance, and psychological resilience
d) Sexual health and reproductive function

Answer: c) Coping strategies, stress tolerance, and psychological resilience

Explanation: The Coping-Stress Tolerance Pattern focuses on evaluating a patient's coping strategies, stress tolerance, and overall psychological resilience in the rehabilitation setting.

109. A rehabilitation nurse notices a patient becoming increasingly anxious about their upcoming discharge. Which of Gordon's Functional Health Patterns should the nurse prioritize in this situation?
a) Sleep-Rest Pattern
b) Cognitive-Perceptual Pattern
c) Coping-Stress Tolerance Pattern
d) Roles-Relationships Pattern

Answer: c) Coping-Stress Tolerance Pattern Explanation: The Coping-Stress Tolerance Pattern is most relevant in this situation, as it focuses on evaluating and addressing a patient's coping strategies, stress tolerance, and psychological resilience in the rehabilitation setting.

110. An appropriate intervention for a patient struggling with stress and anxiety in the rehabilitation setting might include:
a) Encouraging the patient to join a support group
b) Teaching relaxation techniques and stress management strategies
c) Assessing nutritional status and metabolic needs
d) Implementing a personalized exercise program

Answer: b) Teaching relaxation techniques and stress management strategies Explanation: Teaching relaxation techniques and stress management strategies is an appropriate intervention for addressing the Coping-Stress Tolerance Pattern, as it helps patients develop coping skills and improve their stress tolerance and psychological resilience.

111. A patient who has difficulty coping with the emotional impact of their injury may benefit from an intervention focusing on which of Gordon's Functional Health Patterns?
a) Health Perception-Health Management Pattern
b) Nutritional-Metabolic Pattern
c) Roles-Relationships Pattern
d) Coping-Stress Tolerance Pattern

Answer: d) Coping-Stress Tolerance Pattern

Explanation: A patient who struggles with the emotional impact of their injury may benefit from an intervention focusing on the Coping-Stress Tolerance Pattern, which addresses coping strategies, stress tolerance, and psychological resilience in the rehabilitation setting.

112. Which assessment tool would be most helpful for a rehabilitation nurse to evaluate a patient's Coping-Stress Tolerance Pattern?
a) A standardized social support questionnaire
b) A sleep quality and rest habits questionnaire
c) A cognitive abilities and sensory-perceptual function screening test
d) A coping strategies and stress tolerance questionnaire

Answer: d) A coping strategies and stress tolerance questionnaire

Explanation: A coping strategies and stress tolerance questionnaire is the most appropriate assessment tool for evaluating a patient's Coping-Stress Tolerance Pattern, as it helps identify the patient's coping strategies, stress tolerance, and overall psychological resilience in the rehabilitation setting.

113. In the context of rehabilitation nursing, the Value-Belief Pattern primarily focuses on understanding a patient's:
a) Coping strategies and stress tolerance
b) Cultural, spiritual, and personal values and beliefs
c) Nutritional status and metabolic needs
d) Social functioning and support systems

Answer: b) Cultural, spiritual, and personal values and beliefs

Explanation: The Value-Belief Pattern is centered on understanding a patient's cultural, spiritual, and personal values and beliefs that may influence their rehabilitation experience.

114. A rehabilitation nurse is caring for a patient who prefers to use traditional healing practices rather than prescribed medications. Which of Gordon's Functional Health Patterns should the nurse prioritize when addressing this preference?
a) Nutritional-Metabolic Pattern
b) Cognitive-Perceptual Pattern
c) Coping-Stress Tolerance Pattern
d) Value-Belief Pattern

Answer: d) Value-Belief Pattern

Explanation: The Value-Belief Pattern is most relevant in this situation, as it focuses on understanding and respecting a patient's cultural, spiritual, and personal values and beliefs that may influence their rehabilitation experience, including preferences for traditional healing practices.

115 Which intervention would be most helpful for a rehabilitation nurse to address a patient's spiritual needs as part of the Value-Belief Pattern?
a) Offering the patient access to a dietician for nutritional counseling
b) Arranging a visit from a spiritual advisor or chaplain
c) Implementing a personalized exercise program
d) Teaching the patient relaxation techniques and stress management strategies

Answer: b) Arranging a visit from a spiritual advisor or chaplain

Explanation: Arranging a visit from a spiritual advisor or chaplain is an appropriate intervention for addressing a patient's spiritual needs within the Value-Belief Pattern, as it respects and supports the patient's cultural, spiritual, and personal values and beliefs in the rehabilitation setting.

116. When caring for a diverse group of patients, which of Gordon's Functional Health Patterns should a rehabilitation nurse prioritize to ensure culturally competent care?
a) Health Perception-Health Management Pattern
b) Nutritional-Metabolic Pattern
c) Roles-Relationships Pattern
d) Value-Belief Pattern

Answer: d) Value-Belief Pattern

Explanation: The Value-Belief Pattern is most relevant when providing culturally competent care, as it emphasizes understanding and respecting a patient's cultural, spiritual, and personal values and beliefs that may influence their rehabilitation experience.

117. A rehabilitation nurse is working with a patient who is refusing a specific intervention due to religious reasons. Which of the following should the nurse do first to address the patient's concerns?
a) Respect the patient's decision and explore alternative interventions
b) Attempt to persuade the patient to accept the intervention
c) Consult the patient's family members for advice
d) Ignore the patient's concerns and proceed with the intervention

Answer: a) Respect the patient's decision and explore alternative interventions

Explanation: Respecting the patient's decision and exploring alternative interventions is the most appropriate response, as it demonstrates respect for the patient's cultural, spiritual, and personal values and beliefs in line with the Value-Belief Pattern.

118. In a rehabilitation setting, a patient who has recently undergone knee surgery is experiencing difficulty with mobility. Which Functional Health Pattern should the rehabilitation nurse prioritize in creating an individualized care plan for this patient?
a) Nutritional-Metabolic Pattern
b) Activity-Exercise Pattern
c) Cognitive-Perceptual Pattern
d) Sleep-Rest Pattern

Answer: b) Activity-Exercise Pattern

Explanation: The Activity-Exercise Pattern focuses on a patient's functional abilities, mobility, and exercise tolerance. In this case, the rehabilitation nurse should prioritize this pattern to address the patient's mobility issues following knee surgery.

119. A rehabilitation nurse is assessing a patient with a traumatic brain injury. The nurse finds that the patient has difficulty with memory, concentration, and communication. Which Functional Health Pattern is most relevant for developing an appropriate care plan?
a) Health Perception-Health Management Pattern
b) Cognitive-Perceptual Pattern
c) Self-Perception-Self-Concept Pattern
d) Roles-Relationships Pattern

Answer: b) Cognitive-Perceptual Pattern

Explanation: The Cognitive-Perceptual Pattern focuses on a patient's cognitive abilities, sensory-perceptual function, and communication skills. In this case, the rehabilitation nurse should prioritize this pattern to address the patient's cognitive and communication issues following a traumatic brain injury.

120. A patient in a rehabilitation setting has been experiencing poor sleep quality and frequent nighttime awakenings. Which intervention aligns with the Sleep-Rest Pattern to improve the patient's sleep?
a) Providing nutritional counseling to improve the patient's diet
b) Encouraging the patient to participate in social activities
c) Implementing a consistent bedtime routine and sleep environment
d) Teaching the patient relaxation techniques for stress management

Answer: c) Implementing a consistent bedtime routine and sleep environment

Explanation: The Sleep-Rest Pattern focuses on a patient's sleep quality, rest habits, and overall energy levels. Implementing a consistent bedtime routine and sleep environment is an appropriate intervention to address the patient's sleep issues in line with this pattern.

121. A rehabilitation nurse is working with a patient who has recently experienced a stroke and is struggling to adapt to new limitations. Which Functional Health Pattern should the nurse prioritize to address the patient's emotional well-being?
a) Elimination Pattern
b) Self-Perception-Self-Concept Pattern
c) Sexuality-Reproductive Pattern
d) Coping-Stress Tolerance Pattern

Answer: b) Self-Perception-Self-Concept Pattern

Explanation: The Self-Perception-Self-Concept Pattern focuses on a patient's self-image, self-esteem, and emotional well-being. In this case, the rehabilitation nurse should prioritize this pattern to address the patient's emotional well-being as they adapt to new limitations following a stroke.

122. A patient with a spinal cord injury is experiencing challenges in maintaining their role as a parent and partner. Which Functional Health Pattern should the rehabilitation nurse focus on to support the patient's social functioning and adaptation to their new circumstances?
a) Nutritional-Metabolic Pattern
b) Roles-Relationships Pattern
c) Value-Belief Pattern
d) Coping-Stress Tolerance Pattern

Answer: b) Roles-Relationships Pattern
Explanation: The Roles-Relationships Pattern focuses on a patient's social functioning, support systems, and ability to maintain or adapt to their roles. In this case, the rehabilitation nurse should prioritize this pattern to address the patient's challenges in maintaining their role as a parent and partner following a spinal cord injury.

123. A 68-year-old patient with a history of stroke has been admitted to a rehabilitation facility. The patient is experiencing difficulty swallowing, which is affecting their nutritional intake. Which functional health pattern should the nurse prioritize when assessing and addressing this patient's needs?
a) Health Perception-Health Management Pattern
b) Nutritional-Metabolic Pattern
c) Sleep-Rest Pattern
d) Activity-Exercise Pattern

Answer: b) Nutritional-Metabolic Pattern
Rationale: The Nutritional-Metabolic Pattern focuses on the patient's nutritional status and metabolic needs. In this case, the patient's difficulty swallowing is directly affecting their nutritional intake, making this pattern the priority for assessment and intervention.

124. A 45-year-old patient who recently underwent a hip replacement surgery is having trouble adjusting to their temporary mobility limitations. Which functional health pattern should the nurse primarily focus on to help the patient cope with these changes?
a) Self-Perception-Self-Concept Pattern
b) Roles-Relationships Pattern
c) Activity-Exercise Pattern
d) Coping-Stress Tolerance Pattern

Answer: a) Self-Perception-Self-Concept Pattern
Rationale: The Self-Perception-Self-Concept Pattern deals with the patient's self-image, self-esteem, and emotional well-being. Addressing this pattern will help the patient cope with their temporary mobility limitations and adapt to their situation.

125. A patient with a spinal cord injury is admitted to a rehabilitation facility. The patient is experiencing depression and feels isolated from their support system. Which functional health pattern should the nurse prioritize to address these concerns?
a) Cognitive-Perceptual Pattern
b) Self-Perception-Self-Concept Pattern
c) Roles-Relationships Pattern
d) Coping-Stress Tolerance Pattern

Answer: c) Roles-Relationships Pattern
Rationale: The Roles-Relationships Pattern focuses on the patient's social functioning, support systems, and their ability to maintain or adapt to their roles. In this case, addressing the patient's feeling of isolation and connecting them with their support system is a priority.

126. A 57-year-old patient with a traumatic brain injury is admitted to a rehabilitation facility. The patient has difficulty remembering new information and following simple instructions. Which functional health pattern should the nurse focus on when planning interventions for this patient?
a) Cognitive-Perceptual Pattern
b) Sleep-Rest Pattern
c) Value-Belief Pattern
d) Activity-Exercise Pattern

Answer: a) Cognitive-Perceptual Pattern
Rationale: The Cognitive-Perceptual Pattern assesses the patient's cognitive abilities, sensory-perceptual function, and communication skills. In this case, the patient's memory and ability to follow instructions are affected, making this pattern the priority for intervention planning.

127. A patient with a recent below-the-knee amputation is experiencing phantom limb pain. The patient is hesitant to engage in activities and exercises that may help alleviate their pain due to their cultural beliefs. Which functional health pattern should the nurse consider when planning culturally appropriate interventions for this patient?
a) Elimination Pattern
b) Sleep-Rest Pattern
c) Sexuality-Reproductive Pattern
d) Value-Belief Pattern

Answer: d) Value-Belief Pattern
Rationale: The Value-Belief Pattern focuses on understanding the patient's cultural, spiritual, and personal values and beliefs that may influence their rehabilitation experience. In this case, the nurse should consider the patient's cultural beliefs when planning interventions to address phantom limb pain.

128. The rehabilitation nursing process is a systematic method used to guide patient-centered care in the rehabilitation setting. Which of the following is NOT one of the core components of the rehabilitation nursing process?
a) Assessment
b) Diagnosis
c) Medication Administration
d) Evaluation

Answer: c) Medication Administration
Rationale: The core components of the rehabilitation nursing process include assessment, diagnosis, planning, implementation, and evaluation. Medication administration is an aspect of the implementation phase but is not considered a core component on its own.

129. Which of the following best describes the primary purpose of the assessment phase in the rehabilitation nursing process?
a) To identify the patient's strengths and limitations
b) To develop a comprehensive care plan
c) To implement interventions tailored to the patient's needs
d) To evaluate the effectiveness of interventions and modify the care plan as needed

Answer: a) To identify the patient's strengths and limitations
Rationale: During the assessment phase, the nurse gathers information about the patient's physical, psychological, and social functioning. This helps identify the patient's strengths, limitations, and areas requiring intervention.

130. In the rehabilitation nursing process, the diagnosis phase involves:
a) Gathering data about the patient's health status
b) Identifying the patient's actual or potential health problems
c) Developing a plan of care with specific goals and interventions
d) Implementing the care plan and monitoring the patient's progress

Answer: b) Identifying the patient's actual or potential health problems
Rationale: The diagnosis phase of the rehabilitation nursing process involves analyzing the assessment data to identify actual or potential health problems that the patient is experiencing. This information is then used to develop the patient's plan of care.

131. When planning care for a patient in a rehabilitation setting, it is essential to involve the patient and their family in the process. Which of the following best explains the rationale behind this approach?
a) To reduce the workload of the nursing staff
b) To comply with legal and ethical guidelines
c) To ensure the care plan is patient-centered and addresses the patient's unique needs
d) To delegate responsibility for the patient's care to their family

Answer: c) To ensure the care plan is patient-centered and addresses the patient's unique needs
Rationale: Involving the patient and their family in the planning process ensures that the care plan is tailored to the patient's unique needs, preferences, and goals. This promotes patient-centered care and improves the likelihood of successful rehabilitation outcomes.

132. In the context of the rehabilitation nursing process, the evaluation phase is essential for:
a) Identifying the patient's strengths and limitations
b) Formulating nursing diagnoses
c) Planning and implementing interventions
d) Assessing the effectiveness of interventions and modifying the care plan as needed

Answer: d) Assessing the effectiveness of interventions and modifying the care plan as needed
Rationale: The evaluation phase involves assessing the patient's progress toward achieving their goals and determining the effectiveness of the implemented interventions. If necessary, the care plan is modified based on the evaluation findings to better address the patient's needs.

133. In rehabilitation nursing, comprehensive patient assessments are crucial for several reasons. Which of the following is NOT a primary purpose of conducting a thorough patient assessment in rehabilitation nursing?
a) Identifying patients' strengths and limitations
b) Developing a personalized care plan
c) Monitoring the patient's progress in real-time
d) Establishing a baseline for evaluating the effectiveness of interventions

Answer: c) Monitoring the patient's progress in real-time
Rationale: Patient assessments in rehabilitation nursing are essential for identifying patients' strengths and limitations, developing a personalized care plan, and establishing a baseline for evaluating the effectiveness of interventions. Monitoring the patient's progress in real-time is an ongoing process throughout the care delivery but not a primary purpose of the initial assessment.

134. Which of the following standardized assessment tools is most commonly used to evaluate a patient's functional independence in rehabilitation nursing?
a) Barthel Index
b) Mini-Mental State Examination (MMSE)
c) Functional Independence Measure (FIM)
d) Braden Scale for Predicting Pressure Sore Risk

Answer: c) Functional Independence Measure (FIM)
Rationale: The Functional Independence Measure (FIM) is a widely used standardized assessment tool in rehabilitation nursing, specifically designed to evaluate a patient's functional independence in activities of daily living.

135. During the assessment phase in rehabilitation nursing, it is essential to gather information from multiple sources. Which of the following is NOT a recommended source of information for a comprehensive patient assessment?
a) Patient interviews
b) Family and caregiver reports
c) Medical records
d) Previous rehabilitation providers' opinions

Answer: d) Previous rehabilitation providers' opinions
Rationale: While it may be helpful to consult with previous rehabilitation providers, their opinions should not be considered a primary source of information for a comprehensive patient assessment. Patient interviews, family and caregiver reports, and medical records are essential sources of information for a complete assessment.

136. When assessing a patient in a rehabilitation setting, the nurse should consider the patient's individual needs and goals. Which of the following aspects is LEAST important to consider during this process?
a) Patient's preferred learning style
b) Patient's cultural background
c) Patient's favorite color
d) Patient's functional abilities

Answer: c) Patient's favorite color
Rationale: While it is essential to consider various factors when assessing a patient in a rehabilitation setting, the patient's favorite color is not a crucial aspect. Instead, the focus should be on the patient's learning style, cultural background, and functional abilities.

137. Why is it important for rehabilitation nurses to use standardized assessment tools during the assessment phase?
a) Standardized tools allow for a quicker assessment process
b) Standardized tools provide a common language for interdisciplinary communication
c) Standardized tools are legally required in all rehabilitation settings
d) Standardized tools are always more accurate than non-standardized assessments

Answer: b) Standardized tools provide a common language for interdisciplinary communication
Rationale: Using standardized assessment tools is crucial in rehabilitation nursing because they provide a common language for interdisciplinary communication, allowing for better collaboration among the care team. Additionally, standardized tools facilitate comparison of patient outcomes and progress across different settings and time points.

138. Which of the following is a primary purpose of formulating nursing diagnoses in rehabilitation nursing?
a) To provide a comprehensive list of potential patient problems
b) To identify the nurse's personal goals for the patient
c) To classify and prioritize patient concerns based on their impact on rehabilitation outcomes
d) To make a medical diagnosis for the patient

Answer: c) To classify and prioritize patient concerns based on their impact on rehabilitation outcomes
Rationale: The primary purpose of formulating nursing diagnoses in rehabilitation nursing is to classify and prioritize patient concerns based on their impact on rehabilitation outcomes. This allows the care team to focus on addressing the most significant issues and tailor interventions accordingly.

139. Accurate nursing diagnoses in rehabilitation nursing are essential for which of the following reasons?
a) They help minimize patient complaints
b) They reduce the workload of other healthcare professionals
c) They facilitate the development of targeted, patient-centered care plans
d) They make it easier to document the nursing process

Answer: c) They facilitate the development of targeted, patient-centered care plans
Rationale: Accurate nursing diagnoses are essential in rehabilitation nursing because they facilitate the development of targeted, patient-centered care plans. By accurately identifying and prioritizing patient concerns, nurses can tailor interventions to address specific needs and optimize rehabilitation outcomes.

140. In the context of rehabilitation nursing, which of the following is an essential aspect of the nursing diagnosis process?
a) Relying solely on patient-reported information
b) Incorporating interdisciplinary collaboration and input
c) Formulating diagnoses based on the nurse's intuition
d) Focusing on a single aspect of the patient's condition

Answer: b) Incorporating interdisciplinary collaboration and input
Rationale: Incorporating interdisciplinary collaboration and input is essential when formulating nursing diagnoses in rehabilitation nursing. This approach ensures a comprehensive understanding of the patient's needs, fosters effective communication among team members, and facilitates the development of a well-coordinated care plan.

141. What is a critical step in the process of prioritizing nursing diagnoses in rehabilitation nursing?
a) Sorting diagnoses alphabetically
b) Ranking diagnoses based on the nurse's personal preferences
c) Evaluating the potential impact of each diagnosis on the patient's rehabilitation outcomes
d) Prioritizing diagnoses based on the patient's age

Answer: c) Evaluating the potential impact of each diagnosis on the patient's rehabilitation outcomes
Rationale: When prioritizing nursing diagnoses in rehabilitation nursing, it is crucial to evaluate the potential impact of each diagnosis on the patient's rehabilitation outcomes. This process helps determine which concerns are most critical to address and tailor the care plan to maximize the patient's recovery.

142. Which of the following actions should rehabilitation nurses take to ensure accurate nursing diagnoses?
a) Rely on a single assessment tool to gather information
b) Use only patient-reported information when formulating diagnoses
c) Engage in ongoing professional development and education to enhance diagnostic skills
d) Ignore input from other healthcare professionals in the diagnostic process

Answer: c) Engage in ongoing professional development and education to enhance diagnostic skills
Rationale: Rehabilitation nurses should engage in ongoing professional development and education to enhance their diagnostic skills and ensure accurate nursing diagnoses. This approach helps nurses stay current with best practices, evidence-based interventions, and assessment techniques, leading to more accurate diagnoses and better patient outcomes.

143. Which of the following is a key characteristic of a well-formulated rehabilitation nursing care plan?
a) It is based solely on the nurse's perspective and expertise
b) It sets lofty, aspirational goals for the patient
c) It contains generic, non-specific goals that can apply to any patient
d) It is individualized, focusing on the specific needs and goals of the patient

Answer: d) It is individualized, focusing on the specific needs and goals of the patient
Rationale: A well-formulated rehabilitation nursing care plan is individualized, focusing on the specific needs and goals of the patient. This approach ensures that the care plan addresses the unique concerns of each patient and is tailored to promote optimal rehabilitation outcomes.

144. When setting goals for a patient in rehabilitation nursing, it is essential to ensure that goals are:
a) Vague and open-ended
b) Realistic, measurable, and time-bound
c) Based on the nurse's preferences rather than the patient's needs
d) Unrelated to the patient's rehabilitation process

Answer: b) Realistic, measurable, and time-bound. Rationale: When setting goals for a patient in rehabilitation nursing, it is essential to ensure that they are realistic, measurable, and time-bound. This approach helps to promote achievable outcomes, track progress, and adjust the care plan as needed to optimize the patient's rehabilitation journey.

145. Why is interdisciplinary teamwork critical in the planning phase of rehabilitation nursing?
a) It allows nurses to delegate tasks to other team members
b) It facilitates a comprehensive understanding of the patient's needs and fosters effective communication
c) It reduces the need for specialized nursing knowledge
d) It makes the planning process faster and more efficient

Answer: b) It facilitates a comprehensive understanding of the patient's needs and fosters effective communication
Rationale: Interdisciplinary teamwork is critical in the planning phase of rehabilitation nursing because it facilitates a comprehensive understanding of the patient's needs and fosters effective communication among team members. This collaborative approach ensures that all aspects of the patient's care are considered and helps to develop a well-coordinated care plan.

146. Which of the following is a crucial component of developing individualized care plans in rehabilitation nursing?
a) Establishing goals without considering the patient's preferences and values
b) Collaborating with the patient and their family to identify needs, preferences, and goals
c) Creating a one-size-fits-all care plan that can be used for multiple patients
d) Disregarding input from other healthcare professionals

Answer: b) Collaborating with the patient and their family to identify needs, preferences, and goals
Rationale: A crucial component of developing individualized care plans in rehabilitation nursing is collaborating with the patient and their family to identify needs, preferences, and goals. This patient-centered approach ensures that the care plan is tailored to the unique needs of the patient and promotes a sense of ownership and engagement in the rehabilitation process.

147. In the context of rehabilitation nursing, what is the primary purpose of setting patient-centered goals during the planning phase?
a) To establish benchmarks for evaluating the patient's progress and adjusting the care plan as needed
b) To provide a list of tasks for the nurse to complete during each shift
c) To demonstrate the nurse's expertise and knowledge
d) To reduce the likelihood of patient complaints

Answer: a) To establish benchmarks for evaluating the patient's progress and adjusting the care plan as needed
Rationale: The primary purpose of setting patient-centered goals during the planning phase of rehabilitation nursing is to establish benchmarks for evaluating the patient's progress and adjusting the care plan as needed. This process helps to ensure that interventions are effective, and it facilitates ongoing adaptation of the care plan to optimize rehabilitation outcomes.

148. What is the primary goal of selecting evidence-based interventions in rehabilitation nursing?
a) To impress colleagues with the nurse's knowledge of current research
b) To ensure the interventions are grounded in scientific evidence and proven to be effective
c) To minimize the need for collaboration with other healthcare professionals
d) To simplify the implementation process by using standardized interventions

Answer: b) To ensure the interventions are grounded in scientific evidence and proven to be effective
Rationale: The primary goal of selecting evidence-based interventions in rehabilitation nursing is to ensure that the interventions are grounded in scientific evidence and proven to be effective. This approach helps promote optimal patient outcomes and reduces the likelihood of using ineffective or potentially harmful interventions.

149. During the implementation phase of rehabilitation nursing, what is the importance of tailoring care to patients' needs?
a) It reduces the nurse's workload by streamlining care delivery
b) It enables the nurse to practice a wide range of skills and techniques
c) It promotes patient engagement and ownership in the rehabilitation process
d) It allows the nurse to avoid collaborating with other healthcare professionals

Answer: c) It promotes patient engagement and ownership in the rehabilitation process
Rationale: Tailoring care to patients' needs during the implementation phase of rehabilitation nursing is important because it promotes patient engagement and ownership in the rehabilitation process. When care is personalized and responsive to a patient's unique needs, the patient is more likely to actively participate in their rehabilitation and achieve better outcomes.

150. Which of the following best describes the role of patient and family engagement in the implementation phase of rehabilitation nursing?
a) It is a minor aspect of care that should be addressed only if time permits
b) It is essential for fostering a sense of collaboration and partnership between the patient, their family, and the nursing team
c) It is primarily useful for gathering information about the patient's preferences and values
d) It is an unnecessary burden on the patient and their family, as they should trust the nurse's expertise

Answer: b) It is essential for fostering a sense of collaboration and partnership between the patient, their family, and the nursing team. Rationale: Patient and family engagement is essential during the implementation phase of rehabilitation nursing because it fosters a sense of collaboration and partnership between the patient, their family, and the nursing team. This approach helps to ensure that care is responsive to the patient's needs, preferences, and values, and it promotes a sense of ownership and investment in the rehabilitation process.

151. In the context of rehabilitation nursing, why is it crucial to use a patient-centered approach during the implementation phase?
a) It allows the nurse to delegate tasks more effectively
b) It enhances the patient's satisfaction with care and their overall rehabilitation experience
c) It reduces the need for interdisciplinary collaboration
d) It streamlines documentation and record-keeping

Answer: b) It enhances the patient's satisfaction with care and their overall rehabilitation experience
Rationale: Using a patient-centered approach during the implementation phase of rehabilitation nursing is crucial because it enhances the patient's satisfaction with care and their overall rehabilitation experience. This approach ensures that care is tailored to the patient's unique needs and preferences, leading to better engagement, improved outcomes, and a more positive rehabilitation experience.

152. Which of the following is an essential aspect of implementing evidence-based interventions in rehabilitation nursing?
a) Relying solely on personal experience to guide intervention selection
b) Prioritizing interventions that have been published in prestigious medical journals
c) Adapting interventions to meet the specific needs and preferences of the patient
d) Using only interventions that have been endorsed by pharmaceutical companies

Answer: c) Adapting interventions to meet the specific needs and preferences of the patient

153. Why is ongoing evaluation an essential component of the rehabilitation nursing process?
a) It allows the nurse to demonstrate their expertise in patient care
b) It ensures that the nurse can focus on other aspects of care, such as documentation
c) It enables the nurse to monitor patient progress, reassess goals, and adjust care plans as needed
d) It primarily serves to satisfy the requirements of healthcare administrators and regulators

Answer: c) It enables the nurse to monitor patient progress, reassess goals, and adjust care plans as needed. Rationale: Ongoing evaluation is essential in the rehabilitation nursing process because it enables the nurse to monitor patient progress, reassess goals, and adjust care plans as needed. This ongoing process ensures that care remains responsive to the patient's changing needs and promotes optimal outcomes.

154. What is the primary purpose of reassessing a patient's goals during the evaluation phase of rehabilitation nursing?
a) To provide the nurse with an opportunity to practice their assessment skills
b) To determine whether the goals are still relevant, achievable, and appropriate for the patient's current condition
c) To ensure that the nurse has a clear understanding of the patient's preferences and values
d) To comply with the requirements of insurance providers and healthcare administrators

Answer: b) To determine whether the goals are still relevant, achievable, and appropriate for the patient's current condition
Rationale: The primary purpose of reassessing a patient's goals during the evaluation phase of rehabilitation nursing is to determine whether the goals are still relevant, achievable, and appropriate for the patient's current condition. This process helps to ensure that care remains focused on the patient's needs and fosters a sense of progress and accomplishment.

155. Which of the following is a crucial aspect of adjusting care plans in the evaluation phase of rehabilitation nursing?
a) Making changes based solely on the nurse's intuition and experience
b) Modifying the care plan without consulting the patient or their family
c) Collaborating with interdisciplinary team members to ensure a comprehensive and well-coordinated approach to care
d) Prioritizing the implementation of the newest, most innovative interventions

Answer: c) Collaborating with interdisciplinary team members to ensure a comprehensive and well-coordinated approach to care
Rationale: A crucial aspect of adjusting care plans in the evaluation phase of rehabilitation nursing is collaborating with interdisciplinary team members to ensure a comprehensive and well-coordinated approach to care. This collaboration helps to promote optimal patient outcomes by ensuring that all aspects of care are considered and addressed.

156. How can ongoing evaluation in rehabilitation nursing contribute to improved patient outcomes?
a) By increasing patient satisfaction with the rehabilitation experience
b) By ensuring that care remains responsive to the patient's changing needs and circumstances
c) By reducing the workload of the nurse and other healthcare professionals
d) By streamlining the process of documentation and record-keeping

Answer: b) By ensuring that care remains responsive to the patient's changing needs and circumstances. Rationale: Ongoing evaluation in rehabilitation nursing can contribute to improved patient outcomes by ensuring that care remains responsive to the patient's changing needs and circumstances. This responsiveness promotes patient engagement, fosters a sense of progress, and helps to maximize the effectiveness of interventions.

157. In the context of rehabilitation nursing, what is the primary goal of monitoring patient progress during the evaluation phase?
a) To demonstrate the nurse's competence and expertise to colleagues and supervisors
b) To identify areas of improvement and adjust the care plan to better meet the patient's needs
c) To satisfy the requirements of healthcare administrators and regulators
d) To provide the nurse with an opportunity to practice their assessment skills

Answer: b) To identify areas of improvement and adjust the care plan to better meet the patient's needs.

158. Why is thorough documentation crucial in rehabilitation nursing?
a) It enables the nurse to practice their writing and documentation skills
b) It ensures continuity of care and provides a clear record of the patient's rehabilitation journey
c) It primarily serves to satisfy the requirements of healthcare administrators and regulators
d) It reduces the need for interdisciplinary collaboration and communication

Answer: b) It ensures continuity of care and provides a clear record of the patient's rehabilitation journey
Rationale: Thorough documentation is crucial in rehabilitation nursing because it ensures continuity of care and provides a clear record of the patient's rehabilitation journey. Accurate record-keeping helps to inform future care decisions and promotes effective communication among the interdisciplinary team members.

159. Which of the following best describes the role of effective communication in rehabilitation nursing?
a) It allows the nurse to demonstrate their expertise in patient care
b) It primarily serves to gather information about the patient's preferences and values
c) It fosters collaboration, coordination, and information sharing among the interdisciplinary team members
d) It is an unnecessary burden on the nurse, as they should rely on their expertise and intuition

Answer: c) It fosters collaboration, coordination, and information sharing among the interdisciplinary team members
Rationale: Effective communication in rehabilitation nursing fosters collaboration, coordination, and information sharing among the interdisciplinary team members. This approach helps to ensure that care is comprehensive, well-coordinated, and responsive to the patient's needs, promoting optimal patient outcomes.

160. What is the primary purpose of accurate record-keeping in rehabilitation nursing?
a) To provide a clear and comprehensive record of the patient's care, progress, and outcomes
b) To reduce the need for communication among the interdisciplinary team members
c) To demonstrate the nurse's competence and expertise to colleagues and supervisors
d) To streamline the process of documentation and record-keeping for the nursing team

Answer: a) To provide a clear and comprehensive record of the patient's care, progress, and outcomes
Rationale: The primary purpose of accurate record-keeping in rehabilitation nursing is to provide a clear and comprehensive record of the patient's care, progress, and outcomes. This information is essential for informing future care decisions, promoting effective communication among the interdisciplinary team members, and ensuring continuity of care.

161. How does interdisciplinary collaboration contribute to optimal patient outcomes in rehabilitation nursing?
a) It allows the nurse to delegate tasks more effectively
b) It enables the interdisciplinary team to pool their expertise, resources, and perspectives to provide comprehensive, well-coordinated care
c) It primarily serves to satisfy the requirements of healthcare administrators and regulators
d) It reduces the need for accurate documentation and record-keeping

Answer: b) It enables the interdisciplinary team to pool their expertise, resources, and perspectives to provide comprehensive, well-coordinated care
Rationale: Interdisciplinary collaboration contributes to optimal patient outcomes in rehabilitation nursing by enabling the interdisciplinary team to pool their expertise, resources, and perspectives to provide comprehensive, well-coordinated care. This approach helps to ensure that all aspects of the patient's needs are addressed and promotes a seamless, patient-centered rehabilitation experience.

162. In the context of rehabilitation nursing, what is the primary goal of effective communication among interdisciplinary team members?
a) To demonstrate the nurse's competence and expertise in patient care
b) To ensure that care remains focused on the patient's needs, preferences, and values
c) To satisfy the requirements of healthcare administrators and regulators
d) To provide the nurse with an opportunity to practice their communication skills

Answer: b) To ensure that care remains focused on the patient's needs, preferences, and values
Rationale: The primary goal of effective communication among interdisciplinary team members in rehabilitation nursing is to ensure that care remains focused on the patient's needs, preferences, and values.

163. In the context of rehabilitation nursing, what is the primary purpose of respecting patient autonomy?
a) To ensure that the nurse maintains control over the rehabilitation process
b) To uphold the patient's right to make informed decisions about their own care and treatment
c) To primarily serve the requirements of healthcare administrators and regulators
d) To enable the nurse to delegate tasks more effectively

Answer: b) To uphold the patient's right to make informed decisions about their own care and treatment
Rationale: Respecting patient autonomy in rehabilitation nursing is essential to uphold the patient's right to make informed decisions about their own care and treatment. This approach promotes patient-centered care, encourages patient engagement, and fosters a sense of ownership and investment in the rehabilitation process.

164. Which ethical principle is most closely associated with doing good or promoting the well-being of the patient in rehabilitation nursing?
a) Autonomy
b) Beneficence
c) Non-maleficence
d) Justice

Answer: b) Beneficence
Rationale: Beneficence is the ethical principle most closely associated with doing good or promoting the well-being of the patient in rehabilitation nursing. This principle guides the nurse to actively seek the best possible outcomes for the patient by selecting evidence-based interventions, tailoring care to individual needs, and promoting patient engagement.

165. In rehabilitation nursing, the ethical principle of non-maleficence is primarily focused on:
a) Ensuring that care remains focused on the patient's needs, preferences, and values
b) Avoiding harm or minimizing the risk of harm to the patient
c) Promoting the well-being of the patient by actively seeking the best possible outcomes
d) Upholding the patient's right to make informed decisions about their own care and treatment

Answer: b) Avoiding harm or minimizing the risk of harm to the patient
Rationale: In rehabilitation nursing, the ethical principle of non-maleficence is primarily focused on avoiding harm or minimizing the risk of harm to the patient. This principle guides the nurse to select interventions that are evidence-based, appropriate for the patient's condition, and unlikely to cause harm or adverse effects.

166. How does the ethical principle of justice apply to decision-making in rehabilitation nursing?
a) It ensures that resources, treatment, and care are allocated fairly and equitably among patients
b) It promotes the well-being of the patient by actively seeking the best possible outcomes
c) It primarily serves the requirements of healthcare administrators and regulators
d) It upholds the patient's right to make informed decisions about their own care and treatment

Answer: a) It ensures that resources, treatment, and care are allocated fairly and equitably among patients
Rationale: The ethical principle of justice applies to decision-making in rehabilitation nursing by ensuring that resources, treatment, and care are allocated fairly and equitably among patients. This principle guides the nurse to consider the needs and circumstances of all patients in their care and to make decisions that promote fairness and equal opportunity for positive outcomes.

167. Which of the following actions best demonstrates the ethical principle of beneficence in rehabilitation nursing?
a) Prioritizing the newest, most innovative interventions regardless of patient preferences
b) Using evidence-based interventions and tailoring care to the individual patient's needs
c) Allocating resources based on the patient's ability to pay for treatment
d) Delegating tasks to other healthcare professionals without considering their expertise

Answer: b) Using evidence-based interventions and tailoring care to the individual patient's needs
Rationale: The action that best demonstrates the ethical principle of beneficence in rehabilitation nursing is using evidence-based interventions and tailoring care to the individual patient's needs.

168. In the context of rehabilitation nursing, why is cultural competence important?
a) To ensure that the nurse is seen as knowledgeable and experienced by their colleagues
b) To provide culturally sensitive care that respects and acknowledges the patient's beliefs, values, and practices
c) To primarily serve the requirements of healthcare administrators and regulators
d) To reduce the need for interdisciplinary collaboration and communication

Answer: b) To provide culturally sensitive care that respects and acknowledges the patient's beliefs, values, and practices
Rationale: Cultural competence is important in rehabilitation nursing because it enables the nurse to provide culturally sensitive care that respects and acknowledges the patient's beliefs, values, and practices. This approach helps to promote patient engagement, foster trust, and ensure that care is responsive to the unique needs and circumstances of diverse patient populations.

169. Which of the following strategies can help a rehabilitation nurse provide culturally sensitive care?
a) Making assumptions about the patient's beliefs, values, and practices based on their appearance
b) Treating all patients the same, regardless of their cultural background
c) Asking open-ended questions to explore the patient's beliefs, values, and practices
d) Relying solely on their own cultural beliefs and values to guide their care decisions

Answer: c) Asking open-ended questions to explore the patient's beliefs, values, and practices
Rationale: Asking open-ended questions to explore the patient's beliefs, values, and practices is a strategy that can help a rehabilitation nurse provide culturally sensitive care. This approach encourages the patient to share their perspectives and experiences, allowing the nurse to better understand and respond to the patient's unique needs and preferences.

170. How does cultural competence in rehabilitation nursing contribute to health equity?
a) By ensuring that the nurse is seen as an expert in their field
b) By providing care that is responsive to the unique needs and circumstances of diverse patient populations
c) By reducing the workload of the nurse and other healthcare professionals
d) By streamlining the process of documentation and record-keeping

Answer: b) By providing care that is responsive to the unique needs and circumstances of diverse patient populations
Rationale: Cultural competence in rehabilitation nursing contributes to health equity by providing care that is responsive to the unique needs and circumstances of diverse patient populations. This approach helps to reduce health disparities, promote patient engagement, and ensure that all patients have equal access to high-quality, patient-centered care.

171. In the context of rehabilitation nursing, what is the primary goal of developing cultural competence?
a) To comply with the requirements of insurance providers and healthcare administrators
b) To ensure that care remains focused on the nurse's own cultural beliefs and values
c) To promote patient engagement, trust, and satisfaction by providing culturally sensitive care
d) To demonstrate the nurse's competence and expertise to colleagues and supervisors

Answer: c) To promote patient engagement, trust, and satisfaction by providing culturally sensitive care. Rationale: The primary goal of developing cultural competence in rehabilitation nursing is to promote patient engagement, trust, and satisfaction by providing culturally sensitive care. This approach helps to ensure that care is responsive to the unique needs and preferences of diverse patient populations and promotes a more inclusive, equitable healthcare experience.

172. Which of the following actions best demonstrates cultural competence in the rehabilitation nursing process?
a) Assuming that all patients share the same cultural beliefs, values, and practices
b) Ignoring the patient's cultural background when making care decisions
c) Collaborating with interdisciplinary team members who have expertise in the patient's cultural background
d) Relying solely on the nurse's own cultural beliefs and values to guide care decisions

Answer: c) Collaborating with interdisciplinary team members who have expertise in the patient's cultural background.

173. What is a key benefit of interprofessional collaboration in the rehabilitation nursing process?
a) Reducing the need for communication and documentation
b) Ensuring that all care decisions are made solely by the nurse
c) Enhancing patient outcomes through a coordinated and comprehensive approach to care
d) Focusing on the expertise of one discipline to the exclusion of others

Answer: c) Enhancing patient outcomes through a coordinated and comprehensive approach to care
Rationale: Interprofessional collaboration in the rehabilitation nursing process is beneficial because it enhances patient outcomes through a coordinated and comprehensive approach to care. By working together, interdisciplinary team members can leverage their unique skills and knowledge to develop and implement more effective care plans that address the full range of the patient's needs.

174. Which of the following strategies is most effective for fostering communication and cooperation among interdisciplinary team members in the rehabilitation nursing process?
a) Encouraging competition and rivalry between team members
b) Assigning tasks without considering the expertise of each team member
c) Holding regular team meetings to discuss patient progress, share information, and coordinate care
d) Keeping information about the patient's condition and treatment plan confidential from other team members

Answer: c) Holding regular team meetings to discuss patient progress, share information, and coordinate care
Rationale: Holding regular team meetings to discuss patient progress, share information, and coordinate care is an effective strategy for fostering communication and cooperation among interdisciplinary team members in the rehabilitation nursing process. Regular meetings facilitate the exchange of ideas and knowledge, promote shared decision-making, and help to ensure that all team members are working together towards common goals.

175. In the context of rehabilitation nursing, what is the primary goal of interprofessional collaboration?
a) To minimize the workload of the nurse and other healthcare professionals
b) To ensure that care remains focused on the preferences and values of the nurse
c) To enhance patient outcomes by leveraging the unique skills and knowledge of interdisciplinary team members
d) To comply with the requirements of insurance providers and healthcare administrators

Answer: c) To enhance patient outcomes by leveraging the unique skills and knowledge of interdisciplinary team members
Rationale: The primary goal of interprofessional collaboration in rehabilitation nursing is to enhance patient outcomes by leveraging the unique skills and knowledge of interdisciplinary team members. This approach helps to ensure that care is comprehensive, coordinated, and responsive to the full range of the patient's needs and preferences.

176. How does interprofessional collaboration in rehabilitation nursing contribute to improved patient satisfaction?
a) By reducing the need for communication and documentation
b) By providing a more comprehensive and coordinated approach to care
c) By focusing on the expertise of one discipline to the exclusion of others
d) By ensuring that all care decisions are made solely by the nurse

Answer: b) By providing a more comprehensive and coordinated approach to care
Rationale: Interprofessional collaboration in rehabilitation nursing contributes to improved patient satisfaction by providing a more comprehensive and coordinated approach to care. By working together, interdisciplinary team members can develop and implement more effective care plans that address the full range of the patient's needs, leading to better patient outcomes and a more satisfying healthcare experience.

177. Which of the following actions best demonstrates interprofessional collaboration in the rehabilitation nursing process?
a) Prioritizing the opinions and expertise of the nurse above all other team members
b) Making care decisions without consulting other members of the interdisciplinary team
c) Involving all relevant team members in the assessment, planning, implementation, and evaluation of the patient's care
d) Assigning tasks to team members without considering their specific expertise or qualifications

Answer: c) Involving all relevant team members in the assessment, planning, implementation, and evaluation of the patient's care.
Rationale: Involving all relevant team members in the assessment, planning, implementation, and evaluation of the patient's care best demonstrates interprofessional collaboration in the rehabilitation nursing process. By actively involving all relevant team members, the interdisciplinary team can leverage their collective expertise and knowledge to develop and implement more effective, comprehensive care plans that address the full range of the patient's needs and preferences. This collaborative approach ultimately leads to better patient outcomes and a more satisfying healthcare experience for all involved.

178. A 68-year-old patient recovering from a stroke has recently been admitted to the rehabilitation center. The interdisciplinary team is collaborating on developing a care plan for the patient. Which aspect of the rehabilitation nursing process is the team currently working on?
a. Assessment
b. Diagnosis
c. Planning
d. Implementation

Answer: c. Planning
Explanation: The interdisciplinary team is working on developing a care plan, which is the planning phase of the rehabilitation nursing process.

179. A patient in the rehabilitation center has shown significant improvement in their mobility and functional independence. The rehabilitation nurse decides to reassess the goals set for the patient and make necessary adjustments. Which step of the rehabilitation nursing process is the nurse performing?
a. Assessment
b. Diagnosis
c. Evaluation
d. Implementation

Answer: c. Evaluation
Explanation: The nurse is monitoring the patient's progress, reassessing goals, and making adjustments as needed, which represents the evaluation phase of the rehabilitation nursing process.

180. The rehabilitation nurse is gathering information about a new patient's medical history, functional abilities, and social support system. Which component of the rehabilitation nursing process is the nurse performing?
a. Assessment
b. Diagnosis
c. Planning
d. Implementation

Answer: a. Assessment
Explanation: The nurse is collecting comprehensive information about the patient, which is part of the assessment phase of the rehabilitation nursing process.

181. A patient with a spinal cord injury is experiencing difficulty adjusting to the new limitations in mobility. The interdisciplinary team decides to involve a psychologist to provide emotional support and coping strategies. Which aspect of the rehabilitation nursing process does this decision represent?
a. Assessment
b. Diagnosis
c. Planning
d. Implementation

Answer: d. Implementation
Explanation: The interdisciplinary team is selecting an evidence-based intervention tailored to the patient's needs, which is part of the implementation phase of the rehabilitation nursing process.

182. A rehabilitation nurse has identified a potential risk of pressure ulcers for a bed-bound patient. The nurse consults with the interdisciplinary team to discuss preventive measures and potential interventions. Which phase of the rehabilitation nursing process does this action represent?
a. Assessment
b. Diagnosis
c. Planning
d. Implementation

Answer: b. Diagnosis
Explanation: The nurse has identified a potential risk and is discussing it with the interdisciplinary team, which is part of the diagnosis phase of the rehabilitation nursing process.

183. The rehabilitation nursing process is a systematic approach to providing patient-centered care. Which of the following is NOT a core component of this process?
a. Assessment
b. Diagnosis
c. Marketing
d. Evaluation

Answer: c. Marketing
Explanation: The rehabilitation nursing process includes assessment, diagnosis, planning, implementation, and evaluation. Marketing is not a component of this process.

184. What is the primary purpose of the rehabilitation nursing process?
a. To improve patient satisfaction with their care
b. To guide nurses in providing patient-centered care
c. To make the nursing profession more efficient
d. To reduce the number of medical errors in the healthcare system

Answer: b. To guide nurses in providing patient-centered care
Explanation: The rehabilitation nursing process is a systematic approach to guide nurses in providing patient-centered care, focusing on the individual needs and goals of each patient.

185. In the rehabilitation nursing process, when does the assessment phase take place?
a. Before any other phases
b. After the diagnosis phase
c. During the planning phase
d. Throughout the entire process

Answer: d. Throughout the entire process
Explanation: Although the assessment phase is typically thought of as the first step, it is essential to recognize that assessment is an ongoing activity that occurs throughout the entire rehabilitation nursing process.

186. Which of the following is a key feature of the rehabilitation nursing process?
a. It is a linear, one-time process.
b. It requires the nurse to work in isolation.
c. It is a dynamic and cyclical process.
d. It relies solely on the nurse's intuition.

Answer: c. It is a dynamic and cyclical process
Explanation: The rehabilitation nursing process is a dynamic and cyclical process that adjusts to the changing needs and goals of the patient during their rehabilitation journey.

187. Why is interdisciplinary collaboration important in the rehabilitation nursing process?
a. It reduces the workload for nurses.
b. It improves patient outcomes by providing comprehensive care.
c. It increases the prestige of the nursing profession.
d. It simplifies the rehabilitation nursing process.

Answer: b. It improves patient outcomes by providing comprehensive care
Explanation: Interdisciplinary collaboration is vital in the rehabilitation nursing process as it ensures comprehensive, holistic care tailored to the patient's needs, ultimately leading to better patient outcomes.

188. What is the primary purpose of conducting a comprehensive assessment in rehabilitation nursing?
a. To ensure that the nurse has enough information to complete paperwork
b. To identify patients' individual needs and goals
c. To satisfy legal requirements for documentation
d. To determine the most efficient course of action for the nurse

Answer: b. To identify patients' individual needs and goals
Explanation: A comprehensive assessment in rehabilitation nursing aims to identify the individual needs and goals of each patient, providing a foundation for developing an individualized care plan.

189. Why is it important to use standardized assessment tools in rehabilitation nursing?
a. They reduce the time required for assessments.
b. They ensure consistency and accuracy in the assessment process.
c. They are required by law in most healthcare settings.
d. They eliminate the need for clinical judgment.

Answer: b. They ensure consistency and accuracy in the assessment process.
Explanation: Standardized assessment tools are important in rehabilitation nursing because they provide consistency and accuracy in the assessment process, ensuring that all relevant information is gathered and recorded.

190. During the assessment phase of rehabilitation nursing, which of the following should be considered?
a. Only the patient's physical condition
b. The patient's physical, emotional, and social needs
c. The patient's financial situation and insurance coverage
d. The opinions of the patient's family members

Answer: b. The patient's physical, emotional, and social needs
Explanation: A comprehensive assessment in rehabilitation nursing should consider the patient's physical, emotional, and social needs to create a holistic understanding of the patient's situation.

191. What is the role of clinical judgment in the assessment phase of rehabilitation nursing?
a. Clinical judgment is unnecessary if standardized assessment tools are used.
b. Clinical judgment plays a minor role in interpreting assessment findings.
c. Clinical judgment is used to determine which assessment tools are appropriate for a specific patient.
d. Clinical judgment is used to prioritize the patient's needs and goals based on the assessment findings.

Answer: d. Clinical judgment is used to prioritize the patient's needs and goals based on the assessment findings.
Explanation: Clinical judgment is essential during the assessment phase of rehabilitation nursing, as it helps prioritize the patient's needs and goals based on the assessment findings.

192 Which of the following is a reason why it is important to involve the patient and their family in the assessment process?
a. It ensures that the patient's preferences and values are considered.
b. It reduces the workload for the nurse.
c. It ensures that the patient's family members are satisfied with the care provided.
d. It is required by law in most healthcare settings.

Answer: a. It ensures that the patient's preferences and values are considered.
Explanation: Involving the patient and their family in the assessment process is important because it ensures that the patient's preferences and values are considered when developing an individualized care plan.

193. Which of the following best describes the process of formulating nursing diagnoses in rehabilitation nursing?
a. Basing diagnoses solely on the patient's medical history
b. Diagnosing only the most obvious patient concerns
c. Analyzing assessment data to identify actual or potential health problems
d. Making diagnoses based on the nurse's personal opinions

Answer: c. Analyzing assessment data to identify actual or potential health problems
Explanation: The process of formulating nursing diagnoses in rehabilitation nursing involves analyzing the assessment data to identify actual or potential health problems, which can then be addressed through an individualized care plan.

194. Why is it essential to prioritize patient concerns when formulating nursing diagnoses in rehabilitation nursing?
a. To manage the patient's expectations
b. To allocate limited resources efficiently
c. To ensure that the most pressing issues are addressed first
d. To make the diagnostic process easier for the nurse

Answer: c. To ensure that the most pressing issues are addressed first
Explanation: Prioritizing patient concerns is essential in rehabilitation nursing because it ensures that the most pressing issues are addressed first, allowing for the most effective use of resources and the best possible patient outcomes.

195. What is the role of interdisciplinary collaboration in formulating nursing diagnoses in rehabilitation nursing?
a. To reduce the nurse's workload by sharing responsibilities
b. To ensure that all relevant healthcare professionals are aware of the patient's needs
c. To satisfy legal requirements for collaboration
d. To eliminate the need for clinical judgment

Answer: b. To ensure that all relevant healthcare professionals are aware of the patient's needs
Explanation: Interdisciplinary collaboration plays a crucial role in formulating nursing diagnoses in rehabilitation nursing because it ensures that all relevant healthcare professionals are aware of the patient's needs, leading to better care coordination and improved patient outcomes.

196. Which of the following is a potential consequence of inaccurate nursing diagnoses in rehabilitation nursing?
a. Unnecessary interventions
b. Reduced patient satisfaction
c. Increased healthcare costs
d. All of the above

Answer: d. All of the above. Explanation: Inaccurate nursing diagnoses in rehabilitation nursing can lead to unnecessary interventions, reduced patient satisfaction, and increased healthcare costs, making it crucial to ensure that diagnoses are as accurate as possible.

197. When formulating nursing diagnoses in rehabilitation nursing, which of the following should be considered?
a. The patient's medical history
b. The patient's personal preferences and values
c. The input of other healthcare professionals
d. All of the above

Answer: d. All of the above
Explanation: When formulating nursing diagnoses in rehabilitation nursing, it is important to consider the patient's medical history, personal preferences and values, and the input of other healthcare professionals to ensure that the diagnoses are accurate, relevant, and patient-centered.

198. What is the primary purpose of developing individualized care plans for patients in rehabilitation nursing?
a. To standardize care across all patients
b. To ensure that the patient's insurance will cover the treatment
c. To provide a structured framework for patient-centered care
d. To make the nurse's job easier

Answer: c. To provide a structured framework for patient-centered care
Explanation: The primary purpose of developing individualized care plans in rehabilitation nursing is to provide a structured framework for patient-centered care, ensuring that the patient's unique needs, goals, and preferences are taken into account.

199. Why is it important to set realistic goals when developing individualized care plans for patients in rehabilitation nursing?
a. To prevent patient disappointment and maintain motivation
b. To make it easier to achieve the goals
c. To minimize the need for ongoing evaluation
d. To reduce the amount of documentation required

Answer: a. To prevent patient disappointment and maintain motivation
Explanation: Setting realistic goals is important because it helps prevent patient disappointment and maintains motivation by ensuring that the goals are achievable within a reasonable timeframe.

200. In the context of developing individualized care plans for patients in rehabilitation nursing, what does it mean for a goal to be measurable?
a. It can be easily quantified using standardized assessment tools
b. It has a clear endpoint or target that can be observed
c. It can be directly linked to a specific intervention
d. It is achievable within the patient's current resources

Answer: b. It has a clear endpoint or target that can be observed
Explanation: A measurable goal has a clear endpoint or target that can be observed, making it easier to determine whether the goal has been met or if adjustments to the care plan are necessary.

201. Which of the following best describes the role of interdisciplinary teamwork in the planning phase of rehabilitation nursing?
a. To ensure that all healthcare professionals involved in the patient's care are working towards the same goals
b. To delegate tasks and responsibilities among team members
c. To provide an opportunity for team building and professional development
d. To minimize the need for communication between healthcare professionals

Answer: a. To ensure that all healthcare professionals involved in the patient's care are working towards the same goals
Explanation: Interdisciplinary teamwork is crucial in the planning phase of rehabilitation nursing to ensure that all healthcare professionals involved in the patient's care are working towards the same goals, leading to better care coordination and improved patient outcomes.

202. When developing an individualized care plan for a patient in rehabilitation nursing, which of the following factors should be considered?
a. The patient's medical history and current health status
b. The patient's personal preferences, values, and goals
c. The input of other healthcare professionals involved in the patient's care
d. All of the above

Answer: d. All of the above
Explanation: When developing an individualized care plan for a patient in rehabilitation nursing, it is important to consider the patient's medical history and current health status, personal preferences, values, and goals, as well as the input of other healthcare professionals involved in the patient's care. This ensures that the care plan is comprehensive, relevant, and patient-centered.

203. Why is it important for rehabilitation nurses to select evidence-based interventions during the implementation phase?
a. To ensure consistency in the nursing process
b. To increase the likelihood of positive patient outcomes
c. To minimize the need for documentation
d. To make it easier to communicate with other healthcare professionals

Answer: b. To increase the likelihood of positive patient outcomes
Explanation: Selecting evidence-based interventions is important because it increases the likelihood of positive patient outcomes. Evidence-based interventions are supported by scientific research and have been shown to be effective in addressing specific patient needs and goals.

204. How can rehabilitation nurses tailor care to patients' individual needs during the implementation phase?
a. By providing the same interventions to all patients regardless of their unique circumstances
b. By adhering strictly to standardized care plans without considering patient preferences
c. By adjusting interventions based on the patient's response and progress
d. By focusing only on the physical aspects of rehabilitation

Answer: c. By adjusting interventions based on the patient's response and progress
Explanation: Tailoring care to patients' individual needs involves adjusting interventions based on the patient's response and progress. This enables the rehabilitation nurse to provide personalized care that is responsive to the patient's unique circumstances, preferences, and goals.

205. In what way does engaging patients and their families in the care process contribute to the implementation phase of rehabilitation nursing?
a. It ensures that the patient and their family understand and are committed to the care plan
b. It reduces the workload of the rehabilitation nurse
c. It guarantees that the patient will achieve their goals
d. It eliminates the need for interdisciplinary collaboration

Answer: a. It ensures that the patient and their family understand and are committed to the care plan
Explanation: Engaging patients and their families in the care process helps ensure that they understand and are committed to the care plan. This can lead to better adherence to the plan, more effective communication, and ultimately, better patient outcomes.

206. Which of the following best describes the role of patient education during the implementation phase of rehabilitation nursing?
a. To provide information on the patient's diagnosis and prognosis
b. To teach the patient and their family about the care plan and interventions
c. To ensure that the patient understands their rights and responsibilities
d. All of the above

Answer: d. All of the above
Explanation: Patient education during the implementation phase of rehabilitation nursing involves providing information on the patient's diagnosis and prognosis, teaching the patient and their family about the care plan and interventions, and ensuring that the patient understands their rights and responsibilities. This helps promote patient engagement, adherence, and ultimately, better outcomes.

207. Which of the following is an example of an evidence-based intervention in rehabilitation nursing?
a. A novel treatment approach with no scientific support
b. An intervention that has been used for many years but lacks research evidence
c. An intervention that has been proven effective in randomized controlled trials
d. A therapy chosen based on the nurse's personal preferences

Answer: c. An intervention that has been proven effective in randomized controlled trials
Explanation: Evidence-based interventions are those that have been proven effective in rigorous scientific research, such as randomized controlled trials. These interventions are more likely to lead to positive patient outcomes, making them a crucial component of the implementation phase of rehabilitation nursing.

208. What is the primary purpose of ongoing evaluation in the rehabilitation nursing process?
a. To identify new nursing diagnoses
b. To ensure the patient's care plan remains effective and relevant
c. To reduce the need for interdisciplinary collaboration
d. To minimize the workload of the rehabilitation nurse

Answer: b. To ensure the patient's care plan remains effective and relevant
Explanation: Ongoing evaluation is essential to ensure that the patient's care plan remains effective and relevant to their changing needs, progress, and goals. Through continuous evaluation, rehabilitation nurses can identify areas where adjustments to the care plan may be needed to better support the patient's recovery.

209. Which of the following is an important aspect of monitoring patient progress during the evaluation phase of rehabilitation nursing?
a. Documenting patient responses to interventions
b. Ignoring minor changes in the patient's condition
c. Relying solely on objective data
d. Focusing on the patient's weaknesses rather than their strengths

Answer: a. Documenting patient responses to interventions
Explanation: Documenting patient responses to interventions is an important aspect of monitoring patient progress during the evaluation phase. This information can help rehabilitation nurses determine the effectiveness of the interventions and make necessary adjustments to the care plan.

210. How can reassessing patient goals contribute to the evaluation phase of rehabilitation nursing?
a. By helping to identify areas where the patient has made progress
b. By ensuring that goals remain realistic and achievable given the patient's current condition
c. By providing opportunities to involve the patient and their family in decision-making
d. All of the above

Answer: d. All of the above
Explanation: Reassessing patient goals during the evaluation phase can help identify areas where the patient has made progress, ensure that goals remain realistic and achievable given the patient's current condition, and provide opportunities to involve the patient and their family in decision-making. This contributes to the overall effectiveness of the rehabilitation nursing process.

211. Which of the following best describes the role of interdisciplinary collaboration in the evaluation phase of rehabilitation nursing?
a. To allow rehabilitation nurses to delegate tasks to other team members
b. To gather input from various healthcare professionals to inform adjustments to the care plan
c. To ensure that the rehabilitation nurse maintains control over the patient's care
d. To reduce the need for documentation and communication

Answer: b. To gather input from various healthcare professionals to inform adjustments to the care plan
Explanation: Interdisciplinary collaboration plays a crucial role in the evaluation phase of rehabilitation nursing by gathering input from various healthcare professionals to inform adjustments to the care plan. This collaboration helps ensure that the care plan remains comprehensive and responsive to the patient's unique needs and goals.

212. When should the evaluation phase of the rehabilitation nursing process occur?
a. Only at the beginning of the patient's rehabilitation journey
b. Only after the patient has achieved all of their rehabilitation goals
c. Continuously throughout the patient's rehabilitation journey
d. Only when the patient's condition has worsened

Answer: c. Continuously throughout the patient's rehabilitation journey
Explanation: The evaluation phase should occur continuously throughout the patient's rehabilitation journey. Ongoing evaluation allows rehabilitation nurses to monitor patient progress, reassess goals, and adjust care plans as needed to ensure optimal patient outcomes.

213. Which of the following best describes the purpose of thorough documentation in the rehabilitation nursing process?
a. To reduce the workload of the rehabilitation nurse
b. To ensure that patient information is accurately recorded and easily accessible
c. To minimize the need for interdisciplinary collaboration
d. To replace the need for effective communication

Answer: b. To ensure that patient information is accurately recorded and easily accessible
Explanation: Thorough documentation is essential in the rehabilitation nursing process to ensure that patient information is accurately recorded and easily accessible for all members of the interdisciplinary team. Accurate record-keeping helps promote continuity of care and optimal patient outcomes.

214. In the context of rehabilitation nursing, which of the following is an important aspect of effective communication?
a. Using medical jargon when speaking to patients and their families
b. Focusing on conveying information rather than listening to the patient's concerns
c. Providing clear, concise, and relevant information to patients, families, and other healthcare professionals
d. Withholding information from the interdisciplinary team to maintain control over patient care

Answer: c. Providing clear, concise, and relevant information to patients, families, and other healthcare professionals
Explanation: Effective communication in rehabilitation nursing involves providing clear, concise, and relevant information to patients, families, and other healthcare professionals. This ensures that everyone involved in the patient's care has the necessary information to make informed decisions and provide appropriate care.

215. How does interdisciplinary collaboration contribute to effective communication in the rehabilitation nursing process?
a. By reducing the need for documentation
b. By allowing rehabilitation nurses to delegate tasks to other team members
c. By promoting the sharing of knowledge and expertise among healthcare professionals
d. By encouraging competition among team members

Answer: c. By promoting the sharing of knowledge and expertise among healthcare professionals
Explanation: Interdisciplinary collaboration contributes to effective communication in the rehabilitation nursing process by promoting the sharing of knowledge and expertise among healthcare professionals. This collaboration enables the development of comprehensive, patient-centered care plans that reflect the unique needs and goals of each patient.

216. What is one potential consequence of poor documentation in the rehabilitation nursing process?
a. Improved patient outcomes
b. Increased efficiency in the rehabilitation setting
c. Discontinuity of care and potential negative impact on patient outcomes
d. Enhanced interdisciplinary collaboration

Answer: c. Discontinuity of care and potential negative impact on patient outcomes
Explanation: Poor documentation in the rehabilitation nursing process can lead to discontinuity of care and potential negative impact on patient outcomes. Inaccurate or incomplete records can hinder the ability of healthcare professionals to provide appropriate, evidence-based care and monitor patient progress.

217. Which of the following is an essential component of documentation in the rehabilitation nursing process?
a. Using informal language and abbreviations to save time
b. Including the patient's goals, interventions, and progress in the care plan
c. Relying solely on memory when updating patient records
d. Documenting only major events in the patient's rehabilitation journey

Answer: b. Including the patient's goals, interventions, and progress in the care plan
Explanation: An essential component of documentation in the rehabilitation nursing process is including the patient's goals, interventions, and progress in the care plan. This information helps ensure that all members of the interdisciplinary team have access to up-to-date, accurate information about the patient's care, facilitating effective communication and continuity of care.

218. Patient autonomy is an important ethical principle in the rehabilitation nursing process. Which of the following best exemplifies respect for patient autonomy?
a. Making all decisions on behalf of the patient without consulting them
b. Considering the patient's preferences and involving them in decision-making
c. Ignoring the patient's input in favor of what the healthcare team thinks is best
d. Insisting that the patient follows the care plan without question

Answer: b. Considering the patient's preferences and involving them in decision-making
Explanation: Respecting patient autonomy involves considering the patient's preferences and involving them in decision-making, allowing the patient to maintain control over their own care and make informed decisions based on their values and goals.

219. In the context of rehabilitation nursing, the principle of beneficence refers to:
a. Ensuring fair distribution of resources
b. Avoiding harm to the patient
c. Acting in the best interest of the patient
d. Respecting the patient's right to make decisions about their care

Answer: c. Acting in the best interest of the patient
Explanation: Beneficence is the ethical principle that guides healthcare professionals to act in the best interest of the patient. It involves promoting the patient's well-being and providing appropriate care based on their unique needs and goals.

220. Non-maleficence is an important ethical principle in the rehabilitation nursing process. Which of the following actions best demonstrates adherence to this principle?
a. Administering a treatment that may cause harm without considering potential benefits
b. Providing care without considering the potential risks and benefits
c. Refusing to provide care to a patient due to personal beliefs
d. Weighing the potential risks and benefits of an intervention before proceeding

Answer: d. Weighing the potential risks and benefits of an intervention before proceeding
Explanation: Non-maleficence is the ethical principle of "do no harm." Adherence to this principle involves carefully weighing the potential risks and benefits of an intervention before proceeding, to minimize the potential for harm and ensure the best possible outcome for the patient.

221. The principle of justice in rehabilitation nursing involves:
a. Treating all patients with respect and dignity
b. Ensuring that patients have the right to make decisions about their care
c. Acting in the best interest of the patient
d. Providing fair and equal treatment to all patients

Answer: d. Providing fair and equal treatment to all patients
Explanation: The principle of justice in rehabilitation nursing involves providing fair and equal treatment to all patients, regardless of their background or circumstances. This includes ensuring that resources and care are distributed equitably and that each patient has equal access to appropriate care.

222. Which of the following scenarios best demonstrates an ethical dilemma in the rehabilitation nursing process?
a. A patient with a spinal cord injury requires physical therapy but has limited insurance coverage
b. A rehabilitation nurse is unsure whether to use a new evidence-based intervention
c. A patient with cognitive impairments is unable to express their preferences for care
d. The interdisciplinary team disagrees on the best course of action for a patient

Answer: a. A patient with a spinal cord injury requires physical therapy but has limited insurance coverage
Explanation: An ethical dilemma in the rehabilitation nursing process occurs when two or more ethical principles are in conflict, making it difficult to determine the best course of action. In this scenario, the principles of justice (ensuring equal access to care) and beneficence (acting in the best interest of the patient) may be in conflict due to the patient's limited insurance coverage, presenting a challenge for the healthcare team.

223. Which of the following best describes the concept of cultural competence in rehabilitation nursing?
a. Providing the same care to all patients, regardless of their cultural background
b. Understanding and appreciating cultural differences to provide individualized care
c. Assuming all patients from a certain culture have the same needs and preferences
d. Ignoring cultural differences to focus on the medical aspects of care

Answer: b. Understanding and apprecating cultural differences to provide individualized care
Explanation: Cultural competence in rehabilitation nursing involves understanding and appreciating cultural differences and incorporating this understanding into patient care. By doing so, rehabilitation nurses can provide individualized care that is respectful of each patient's unique cultural background, values, and beliefs.

224. What is the primary goal of providing culturally sensitive care in the rehabilitation nursing process?
a. To avoid offending patients from diverse cultural backgrounds
b. To ensure that all patients receive the same level of care
c. To promote health equity and improve patient outcomes
d. To comply with organizational policies and regulations

Answer: c. To promote health equity and improve patient outcomes
Explanation: The primary goal of providing culturally sensitive care in the rehabilitation nursing process is to promote health equity and improve patient outcomes. By considering and addressing each patient's unique cultural needs, rehabilitation nurses can provide more effective care and help reduce disparities in healthcare.

225. Which of the following strategies can help rehabilitation nurses develop cultural competence?
a. Attending cultural sensitivity training workshops
b. Relying on stereotypes to guide patient care
c. Avoiding conversations about cultural differences
d. Assuming that all patients from a certain culture share the same values and beliefs

Answer: a. Attending cultural sensitivity training workshops
Explanation: Attending cultural sensitivity training workshops can help rehabilitation nurses develop cultural competence by providing information on different cultural practices, beliefs, and values. This knowledge can then be applied in the clinical setting to provide individualized, culturally sensitive care.

226. A rehabilitation nurse is working with a patient whose cultural beliefs conflict with the recommended treatment plan. What is the most appropriate course of action for the nurse?
a. Insist that the patient follow the recommended treatment plan
b. Work with the patient and the interdisciplinary team to develop a mutually acceptable plan
c. Disregard the patient's cultural beliefs and proceed with the original treatment plan
d. Allow the patient to follow their cultural beliefs without offering any alternatives

Answer: b. Work with the patient and the interdisciplinary team to develop a mutually acceptable plan
Explanation: When a patient's cultural beliefs conflict with the recommended treatment plan, it's important for the rehabilitation nurse to collaborate with the patient and the interdisciplinary team to develop a mutually acceptable plan. This approach demonstrates respect for the patient's autonomy and cultural beliefs while ensuring that appropriate care is provided.

227. In order to promote health equity in the rehabilitation nursing process, it is important for nurses to:
a. Provide the same care to all patients, regardless of their cultural background
b. Focus only on the medical aspects of care and avoid discussions about culture
c. Understand and address the unique cultural needs of each patient
d. Rely on generalizations about cultural groups to guide patient care

Answer: c. Understand and address the unique cultural needs of each patient
Explanation: To promote health equity in the rehabilitation nursing process, it's important for nurses to understand and address the unique cultural needs of each patient. By doing so, they can provide individualized, culturally sensitive care that helps to reduce disparities in healthcare and improve patient outcomes.

228. Which of the following best describes the purpose of interprofessional collaboration in the rehabilitation nursing process?
a. To minimize the workload of rehabilitation nurses
b. To ensure a consistent approach to patient care across disciplines
c. To improve patient outcomes by leveraging the expertise of various healthcare professionals
d. To comply with organizational policies and regulations

Answer: c. To improve patient outcomes by leveraging the expertise of various healthcare professionals

Explanation: The primary purpose of interprofessional collaboration in the rehabilitation nursing process is to improve patient outcomes by leveraging the expertise of various healthcare professionals. By working together, interdisciplinary teams can develop and implement comprehensive care plans that address the complex needs of patients in the rehabilitation setting.

229. Which of the following is an essential component of effective interprofessional collaboration?
a. Clear and open communication among team members
b. A hierarchical decision-making process
c. A focus on individual achievements and successes
d. Competitiveness among healthcare professionals

Answer: a. Clear and open communication among team members

Explanation: Clear and open communication is essential for effective interprofessional collaboration. By fostering a culture of transparency and information sharing, interdisciplinary teams can work together more efficiently, address patient needs more effectively, and ultimately improve patient outcomes.

230. A rehabilitation nurse is part of an interdisciplinary team caring for a patient with multiple complex needs. What is the most appropriate strategy for the nurse to ensure effective collaboration with the team?
a. Keep all patient information confidential and share it only with the physician
b. Delegate all decision-making to the team leader
c. Actively participate in team meetings and contribute to discussions about the patient's care
d. Focus solely on nursing interventions, leaving other aspects of care to other team members

Answer: c. Actively participate in team meetings and contribute to discussions about the patient's care

Explanation: To ensure effective collaboration with the interdisciplinary team, the rehabilitation nurse should actively participate in team meetings and contribute to discussions about the patient's care. This approach ensures that the nurse's expertise is integrated into the care plan and allows for a more comprehensive approach to patient care.

231. How can a rehabilitation nurse best foster a positive team dynamic within an interdisciplinary team?
a. By asserting dominance over other team members
b. By focusing on individual achievements rather than team goals
c. By demonstrating respect and valuing the input of all team members
d. By avoiding confrontation and remaining passive in team meetings

Answer: c. By demonstrating respect and valuing the input of all team members
Explanation: Fostering a positive team dynamic within an interdisciplinary team involves demonstrating respect and valuing the input of all team members. By encouraging open communication, listening actively, and acknowledging the expertise of others, the rehabilitation nurse can help create a collaborative environment where all team members feel valued and heard.

232. Which of the following is a key benefit of interprofessional collaboration in the rehabilitation nursing process?
a. Reducing the need for continuing education among healthcare professionals
b. Enhancing the quality and comprehensiveness of patient care
c. Eliminating the need for patient and family involvement in the care process
d. Decreasing the need for evidence-based practice in the rehabilitation setting

Answer: b. Enhancing the quality and comprehensiveness of patient care
Explanation: A key benefit of interprofessional collaboration in the rehabilitation nursing process is enhancing the quality and comprehensiveness of patient care. By working together, interdisciplinary teams can develop and implement care plans that address the complex needs of patients more effectively, ultimately improving patient outcomes.

CASE STUDY

Maria is a 65-year-old woman who recently suffered a stroke, resulting in left-sided weakness and difficulty with speech. She was admitted to a rehabilitation facility where an interdisciplinary team, including a rehabilitation nurse, physical therapist, occupational therapist, and speech therapist, has been assembled to address her needs. The team is following the rehabilitation nursing process to provide Maria with comprehensive, patient-centered care.

233. As part of the assessment phase of the rehabilitation nursing process, which of the following is the most appropriate action for the rehabilitation nurse?
a. Conduct a comprehensive assessment of Maria's physical, cognitive, emotional, and social needs
b. Rely on the physical therapist's assessment of Maria's mobility limitations
c. Focus solely on Maria's difficulty with speech and leave the rest of the assessment to other team members
d. Wait for the occupational therapist to complete their assessment before starting any nursing interventions

Answer: a. Conduct a comprehensive assessment of Maria's physical, cognitive, emotional, and social needs
Explanation: During the assessment phase, the rehabilitation nurse should conduct a comprehensive assessment of Maria's needs, taking into account various aspects of her health and well-being. This will provide the interdisciplinary team with a better understanding of Maria's overall condition and inform the development of a comprehensive care plan.

234. Based on the team's assessment, one of Maria's nursing diagnoses is "Impaired physical mobility related to left-sided weakness." What is the most appropriate goal for addressing this nursing diagnosis during the planning phase?
a. Maria will walk independently without assistance within one day
b. Maria will regain full mobility within a week
c. Maria will demonstrate improved mobility by using a walker with minimal assistance within two weeks
d. Maria will not require any mobility assistance within a month

Answer: c. Maria will demonstrate improved mobility by using a walker with minimal assistance within two weeks
Explanation: When setting goals during the planning phase, it is important to ensure they are realistic, measurable, and patient-centered. In this case, the most appropriate goal is for Maria to demonstrate improved mobility by using a walker with minimal assistance within two weeks. This goal is specific and achievable, taking into account Maria's current limitations and the expected progress during rehabilitation.

235. During the implementation phase, the rehabilitation nurse should:
a. Delegate all mobility interventions to the physical therapist
b. Provide nursing interventions only when Maria requests assistance
c. Select evidence-based interventions tailored to Maria's individual needs and goals
d. Implement a standardized care plan without considering Maria's specific needs

Answer: c. Select evidence-based interventions tailored to Maria's individual needs and goals
Explanation: During the implementation phase, the rehabilitation nurse should select evidence-based interventions tailored to Maria's individual needs and goals. This approach ensures that Maria receives care that is not only supported by current research but also addresses her specific needs and preferences.

236. In order to promote effective interprofessional collaboration, the rehabilitation nurse should:
a. Attend interdisciplinary team meetings and actively contribute to discussions about Maria's care
b. Focus solely on nursing interventions and leave the coordination of care to the team leader
c. Rely on written reports from other team members instead of attending team meetings
d. Assume that other team members are aware of Maria's nursing needs and goals

Answer: a. Attend interdisciplinary team meetings and actively contribute to discussions about Maria's care
Explanation: To promote effective interprofessional collaboration, the rehabilitation nurse should attend interdisciplinary team meetings and actively contribute to discussions about Maria's care. This approach ensures that the nurse's expertise is integrated into the care plan, allowing for a more comprehensive approach to patient care.

237. During the evaluation phase of the rehabilitation nursing process, the rehabilitation nurse should:
a. Focus solely on Maria's progress related to nursing interventions
b. Reassess Maria's goals and adjust the care plan as needed based on her progress and ongoing needs
c. Rely on other team members' evaluations of Maria's progress without conducting their own evaluation
d. Disregard any changes in Maria's condition that may require adjustments to the care plan

Answer: b. Reassess Maria's goals and adjust the care plan as needed based on her progress and ongoing needs
Explanation: During the evaluation phase, the rehabilitation nurse should reassess Maria's goals and adjust the care plan as needed based on her progress and ongoing needs. This ensures that the care provided remains relevant and responsive to Maria's current condition and supports her continued progress toward her rehabilitation goals.

238. . To provide long-term care for patients in a hospital setting
b. To help patients regain their independence and return to their previous roles in society
c. To focus solely on physical recovery, leaving psychosocial aspects to other professionals
d. To support patients' transition from hospital to nursing home care

Answer: b. To help patients regain their independence and return to their previous roles in society
Explanation: The primary goal of community reintegration is to help patients regain their independence and return to their previous roles in society. This involves addressing physical, cognitive, emotional, and social aspects of recovery, and working with an interdisciplinary team to provide comprehensive care tailored to each patient's needs.

239. Which of the following is NOT a key component of community reintegration in the context of rehabilitation nursing?
a. Supporting patients' physical recovery and functional independence
b. Facilitating patients' emotional and psychological well-being
c. Collaborating with an interdisciplinary team to address patients' needs
d. Prioritizing nursing interventions over input from other healthcare professionals

Answer: d. Prioritizing nursing interventions over input from other healthcare professionals
Explanation: Community reintegration in the context of rehabilitation nursing involves collaboration with an interdisciplinary team to address patients' needs. Prioritizing nursing interventions over input from other healthcare professionals is not conducive to successful reintegration, as it undermines the value of teamwork and comprehensive care.

240. How can rehabilitation nurses support patients' emotional and psychological well-being during the community reintegration process?
a. By providing ongoing counseling and therapy sessions
b. By solely focusing on patients' physical recovery
c. By collaborating with mental health professionals to address patients' emotional needs
d. By disregarding patients' feelings and focusing only on objective measures of progress

Answer: c. By collaborating with mental health professionals to address patients' emotional needs
Explanation: Rehabilitation nurses can support patients' emotional and psychological well-being during community reintegration by collaborating with mental health professionals to address their emotional needs. This may involve referrals to therapists, support groups, or other resources that can help patients navigate the challenges of reintegration.

241. Which of the following best describes the role of family and caregivers in the community reintegration process?
a. Family and caregivers should not be involved, as they may impede the patient's progress
b. Family and caregivers play a critical role in providing emotional and practical support to the patient
c. Family and caregivers should only be involved in the physical aspects of the patient's recovery
d. Family and caregivers should handle all aspects of the patient's care without input from healthcare professionals

Answer: b. Family and caregivers play a critical role in providing emotional and practical support to the patient
Explanation: Family and caregivers play a critical role in the community reintegration process by providing emotional and practical support to the patient. They can help reinforce rehabilitation strategies, offer encouragement, and assist with daily activities, all of which contribute to a successful reintegration.

242. Which of the following is an example of a community resource that rehabilitation nurses may connect patients with during the reintegration process?
a. A local gym for physical therapy and exercise
b. A nursing home for long-term care
c. A hospital for inpatient treatment
d. A specialty clinic for acute medical interventions

Answer: a. A local gym for physical therapy and exercise
Explanation: A local gym for physical therapy and exercise is an example of a community resource that rehabilitation nurses may connect patients with during the reintegration process. These resources can help patients continue their recovery, maintain their physical well-being, and build social connections in their community.

243. Which of the following is a common physical barrier to community reintegration for patients undergoing rehabilitation?
a. Lack of social support from friends and family
b. Limited accessibility to public transportation and buildings
c. Difficulty concentrating or making decisions
d. Fear of stigmatization or discrimination

Answer: b. Limited accessibility to public transportation and buildings
Explanation: Limited accessibility to public transportation and buildings is a common physical barrier to community reintegration. This can hinder patients' ability to participate in daily activities, access healthcare services, and engage with their community, making it more difficult to regain independence and return to their previous roles in society.

244. How might cognitive impairments pose a barrier to community reintegration?
a. They may make it difficult for patients to engage in social activities
b. They can cause patients to become physically dependent on others
c. They may affect patients' ability to process information, problem-solve, or communicate effectively
d. They can lead to social isolation due to lack of understanding or empathy from others

Answer: c. They may affect patients' ability to process information, problem-solve, or communicate effectively
Explanation: Cognitive impairments may pose a barrier to community reintegration by affecting patients' ability to process information, problem-solve, or communicate effectively. This can make it challenging for patients to manage daily activities, interact with others, and adapt to new situations, thereby hindering their reintegration process.

245. Which of the following emotional barriers may impact a patient's community reintegration process?
a. Limited access to healthcare services in their community
b. Difficulty navigating public transportation systems
c. Anxiety, depression, or other mental health issues
d. Physical impairments that restrict mobility

Answer: c. Anxiety, depression, or other mental health issues
Explanation: Anxiety, depression, or other mental health issues are emotional barriers that may impact a patient's community reintegration process. These emotional challenges can make it difficult for patients to cope with the changes and challenges associated with reintegration, affecting their motivation and ability to engage in rehabilitation activities and social interactions.

246. Social barriers to community reintegration may include:
a. Unsupportive family or friends
b. Cognitive impairments affecting communication
c. Inaccessible public spaces
d. Difficulty finding appropriate healthcare services

Answer: a. Unsupportive family or friends
Explanation: Unsupportive family or friends can act as a social barrier to community reintegration. Social support is critical during the reintegration process, and a lack of support can hinder patients' emotional well-being, motivation, and overall progress.

247. An environmental factor that may pose a barrier to community reintegration is:
a. Limited availability of specialized healthcare services in the community
b. The patient's level of physical functioning
c. The patient's ability to cope with stress
d. The patient's level of social support from friends and family

Answer: a. Limited availability of specialized healthcare services in the community
Explanation: Limited availability of specialized healthcare services in the community is an environmental factor that may pose a barrier to community reintegration. Patients may struggle to access the services they need, which could affect their recovery, overall health, and ability to reintegrate into their community.

248. When assessing a patient's readiness for community reintegration, it is important to evaluate their physical functioning. Which of the following factors should be considered?
a. The patient's ability to perform activities of daily living independently
b. The patient's level of social support from friends and family
c. The patient's emotional well-being and ability to cope with stress
d. The patient's cognitive abilities, such as memory and problem-solving skills

Answer: a. The patient's ability to perform activities of daily living independently
Explanation: Evaluating a patient's physical functioning involves assessing their ability to perform activities of daily living independently. This includes their mobility, self-care skills, and overall physical capabilities, which can impact their ability to successfully reintegrate into the community.

249. In order to assess a patient's cognitive functioning for community reintegration, a rehabilitation nurse should evaluate:
a. The patient's ability to communicate effectively with others
b. The patient's access to healthcare services in their community
c. The patient's support network and relationships
d. The patient's ability to navigate public transportation systems

Answer: a. The patient's ability to communicate effectively with others
Explanation: Assessing a patient's cognitive functioning involves evaluating their ability to process information, problem-solve, and communicate effectively with others. These skills are crucial for successful community reintegration, as they impact the patient's ability to adapt to new situations, manage daily activities, and interact with others.

250. Which of the following aspects of emotional functioning is crucial to assess when determining a patient's readiness for community reintegration?
a. The patient's level of physical independence
b. The patient's ability to access healthcare services in their community
c. The patient's emotional well-being and ability to cope with stress
d. The patient's relationships with friends and family

Answer: c. The patient's emotional well-being and ability to cope with stress
Explanation: When assessing a patient's emotional functioning, it is crucial to evaluate their emotional well-being and ability to cope with stress. This includes assessing their mental health, resilience, and coping strategies, which can impact their ability to manage challenges and adapt to changes during the reintegration process.

251. When assessing a patient's social functioning for community reintegration, which of the following should be considered?
a. The patient's ability to perform activities of daily living independently
b. The patient's cognitive abilities, such as memory and problem-solving skills
c. The patient's level of social support from friends and family
d. The patient's access to healthcare services in their community

Answer: c. The patient's level of social support from friends and family
Explanation: Assessing a patient's social functioning involves evaluating their level of social support from friends and family, as well as their ability to engage in social activities and maintain relationships. This is important for community reintegration, as a strong support network can help patients navigate challenges, maintain emotional well-being, and achieve their rehabilitation goals.

252. A comprehensive assessment of a patient's readiness for community reintegration should include:
a. Evaluating only the patient's physical and cognitive functioning
b. Focusing solely on the patient's emotional well-being and coping strategies
c. Assessing only the patient's social support network and relationships
d. Evaluating the patient's physical, cognitive, emotional, and social functioning

Answer: d. Evaluating the patient's physical, cognitive, emotional, and social functioning
Explanation: A comprehensive assessment of a patient's readiness for community reintegration should include evaluating their physical, cognitive, emotional, and social functioning. This holistic approach ensures that all factors impacting the patient's ability to successfully reintegrate into the community are considered, and helps to guide the development of individualized care plans that address their unique needs

253. When developing a comprehensive community reintegration plan, which of the following is crucial to ensure the plan is tailored to the patient's unique needs?
a. Relying solely on input from healthcare professionals
b. Setting goals based on the rehabilitation team's priorities
c. Involving the patient and their family in goal-setting and decision-making
d. Focusing only on the patient's physical needs and abilities

Answer: c. Involving the patient and their family in goal-setting and decision-making
Explanation: Involving the patient and their family in goal-setting and decision-making is crucial to ensure that the community reintegration plan is tailored to the patient's unique needs, preferences, and circumstances. This collaborative approach helps to promote patient-centered care and enhance patient engagement in the rehabilitation process.

254. Which of the following best describes the role of interdisciplinary collaboration in developing a community reintegration plan?
a. Interdisciplinary collaboration is not necessary, as rehabilitation nurses can create the plan independently
b. Interdisciplinary collaboration ensures that only one healthcare professional is responsible for the patient's care
c. Interdisciplinary collaboration facilitates the sharing of expertise and resources among healthcare professionals
d. Interdisciplinary collaboration is only important when addressing the patient's physical needs

Answer: c. Interdisciplinary collaboration facilitates the sharing of expertise and resources among healthcare professionals
Explanation: Interdisciplinary collaboration is essential in developing a community reintegration plan, as it facilitates the sharing of expertise and resources among healthcare professionals. This collaborative approach ensures that the plan addresses the patient's diverse needs in a comprehensive and holistic manner, ultimately leading to better patient outcomes.

255. What is a key component of a successful community reintegration plan?
a. Creating a plan that focuses exclusively on the patient's physical needs
b. Setting goals that are vague and difficult to measure
c. Establishing realistic, measurable, and patient-centered goals
d. Excluding the patient's family from the planning process

Answer: c. Establishing realistic, measurable, and patient-centered goals
Explanation: Establishing realistic, measurable, and patient-centered goals is a key component of a successful community reintegration plan. These goals help to ensure that the plan is tailored to the patient's unique needs and preferences, and provide a clear framework for evaluating the patient's progress and adjusting the plan as needed.

256. When creating a community reintegration plan, which of the following should be considered to ensure the plan is comprehensive?
a. Physical, cognitive, emotional, and social functioning
b. Only physical and cognitive functioning
c. Only emotional and social functioning
d. Only physical functioning

Answer: a. Physical, cognitive, emotional, and social functioning
Explanation: When creating a community reintegration plan, it is important to consider the patient's physical, cognitive, emotional, and social functioning. This comprehensive approach ensures that the plan addresses all aspects of the patient's well-being and promotes a successful transition to community living.

257. How can rehabilitation nurses support the implementation of a community reintegration plan?
a. By providing patient and family education on available resources and support services
b. By focusing solely on the patient's physical rehabilitation
c. By delegating all responsibility to the patient and their family
d. By excluding other healthcare professionals from the planning process

Answer: a. By providing patient and family education on available resources and support services
Explanation: Rehabilitation nurses play a critical role in supporting the implementation of a community reintegration plan by providing patient and family education on available resources and support services. This helps to empower patients and their families to actively engage in the rehabilitation process, access necessary resources, and achieve their reintegration goals.

258. Which of the following best describes the primary goal of physical and occupational therapy in community reintegration?
a. To focus solely on restoring the patient's previous level of functioning
b. To develop functional skills and adaptations that promote independence and participation in daily activities
c. To provide only short-term support for patients during their hospital stay
d. To prioritize the physical aspects of rehabilitation over cognitive and emotional factors

Answer: b. To develop functional skills and adaptations that promote independence and participation in daily activities
Explanation: The primary goal of physical and occupational therapy in community reintegration is to develop functional skills and adaptations that promote independence and participation in daily activities. This comprehensive approach helps patients successfully transition back into their communities and engage in meaningful activities that enhance their overall well-being.

259. What is a key role of occupational therapy in preparing patients for successful community reintegration?
a. Assessing and treating only physical impairments
b. Teaching patients how to manage their finances
c. Developing strategies to address cognitive and emotional challenges
d. Providing one-time consultations without ongoing support

Answer: c. Developing strategies to address cognitive and emotional challenges
Explanation: A key role of occupational therapy in preparing patients for successful community reintegration is developing strategies to address cognitive and emotional challenges. Occupational therapists work with patients to improve their problem-solving, memory, and emotional regulation skills, enabling them to better manage daily tasks and participate in their communities.

260. How do physical therapists contribute to community reintegration for patients with mobility impairments?
a. By exclusively focusing on upper body strength
b. By only addressing the patient's physical appearance
c. By helping patients develop the necessary strength, balance, and endurance for mobility
d. By avoiding any adaptations or assistive devices in favor of natural recovery

Answer: c. By helping patients develop the necessary strength, balance, and endurance for mobility
Explanation: Physical therapists contribute to community reintegration for patients with mobility impairments by helping them develop the necessary strength, balance, and endurance for mobility. This includes working with patients on exercises, mobility training, and, if necessary, recommending and training them on the use of assistive devices to promote independence and safety.

261. In the context of community reintegration, which of the following is an important aspect of the collaboration between physical and occupational therapists?
a. Competing to see which discipline can achieve the best patient outcomes
b. Sharing expertise and resources to provide a comprehensive approach to rehabilitation
c. Completely separating their roles, with no overlap or communication
d. Focusing only on their respective areas of expertise, without considering the patient's overall needs

Answer: b. Sharing expertise and resources to provide a comprehensive approach to rehabilitation
Explanation: In the context of community reintegration, an important aspect of the collaboration between physical and occupational therapists is sharing expertise and resources to provide a comprehensive approach to rehabilitation. This interdisciplinary teamwork ensures that the patient's diverse needs are addressed in a holistic manner, ultimately leading to better patient outcomes.

262. Which of the following best exemplifies an adaptive strategy that may be utilized by an occupational therapist to promote community reintegration?
a. Encouraging the patient to avoid any activities that may be challenging
b. Teaching the patient to use adaptive equipment, such as a long-handled reacher, to perform daily tasks
c. Focusing solely on regaining pre-injury skills without considering alternative methods
d. Ignoring cognitive and emotional factors that may impact the patient's ability to reintegrate

Answer: b. Teaching the patient to use adaptive equipment, such as a long-handled reacher, to perform daily tasks.

263. How does psychosocial support contribute to a patient's successful community reintegration?
a. By ignoring emotional and social factors in favor of focusing on physical recovery
b. By promoting the patient's ability to cope with stress and adapt to new circumstances
c. By solely relying on medication to address the patient's emotional needs
d. By discouraging the patient from seeking assistance from support networks

Answer: b. By promoting the patient's ability to cope with stress and adapt to new circumstances
Explanation: Psychosocial support contributes to a patient's successful community reintegration by promoting their ability to cope with stress and adapt to new circumstances. This support helps patients build resilience and develop effective strategies for managing the emotional and social challenges they may face during the reintegration process.

264. Which of the following is a key element of effective stress management in the context of community reintegration?
a. Ignoring stress and hoping it will go away on its own
b. Identifying and addressing sources of stress through problem-solving techniques
c. Relying solely on medication to manage stress
d. Encouraging the patient to avoid any activities that may cause stress

Answer: b. Identifying and addressing sources of stress through problem-solving techniques
Explanation: A key element of effective stress management in the context of community reintegration is identifying and addressing sources of stress through problem-solving techniques. By helping patients recognize their stressors and develop strategies to cope with them, rehabilitation professionals can promote a more successful reintegration process.

265. How can support networks play a role in facilitating community reintegration for patients?
a. By encouraging dependence on others rather than promoting independence
b. By providing emotional support, practical assistance, and resources for the patient
c. By taking over all decision-making for the patient
d. By undermining the patient's confidence and self-efficacy

Answer: b. By providing emotional support, practical assistance, and resources for the patient
Explanation: Support networks play a crucial role in facilitating community reintegration for patients by providing emotional support, practical assistance, and resources. These networks can include family members, friends, healthcare providers, and community organizations, all of which can contribute to the patient's overall well-being and success in reintegrating into their community.

266. What is a key goal of counseling during the community reintegration process?
a. To focus solely on the patient's physical recovery
b. To develop the patient's coping strategies and emotional resilience
c. To encourage the patient to ignore their emotional needs
d. To avoid discussing any challenges the patient may face during reintegration

Answer: b. To develop the patient's coping strategies and emotional resilience
Explanation: A key goal of counseling during the community reintegration process is to develop the patient's coping strategies and emotional resilience. By helping patients understand and manage their emotions, counselors can support their overall well-being and ability to adapt to new circumstances during reintegration.

267. In the context of community reintegration, which of the following is an example of a coping strategy that rehabilitation professionals might encourage patients to adopt?
a. Avoiding any activities that may be emotionally challenging
b. Relying exclusively on medication to manage emotional distress
c. Practicing relaxation techniques, such as deep breathing or mindfulness
d. Suppressing emotions and refusing to discuss any difficulties they may be experiencing

Answer: c. Practicing relaxation techniques, such as deep breathing or mindfulness
Explanation: In the context of community reintegration, practicing relaxation techniques, such as deep breathing or mindfulness, is an example of a coping strategy that rehabilitation professionals might encourage patients to adopt. These techniques can help patients manage stress, anxiety, and other emotional challenges they may face during the reintegration process.

268. Why is vocational rehabilitation important in the context of community reintegration for patients?
a. It focuses on the patient's hobbies rather than their work abilities
b. It contributes to patients' self-esteem and social connections
c. It only addresses patients' short-term employment needs
d. It has no impact on patients' long-term financial stability

Answer: b. It contributes to patients' self-esteem and social connections
Explanation: Vocational rehabilitation is important in the context of community reintegration because it contributes to patients' self-esteem and social connections. By helping patients return to work or find new employment, vocational rehabilitation can enhance their sense of purpose, independence, and well-being.

269. Which of the following is an effective strategy for job training in vocational rehabilitation?
a. Encouraging patients to figure things out on their own without guidance
b. Providing patients with tailored training programs that address their unique needs and abilities
c. Focusing on training for jobs that are unrelated to the patient's interests or abilities
d. Ignoring the need for any adaptations or accommodations in the workplace

Answer: b. Providing patients with tailored training programs that address their unique needs and abilities
Explanation: An effective strategy for job training in vocational rehabilitation is to provide patients with tailored training programs that address their unique needs and abilities. By offering customized training, rehabilitation professionals can better prepare patients for successful employment and community reintegration.

270. How can workplace accommodations support patients in successfully reintegrating into their community?
a. By eliminating the need for any ongoing rehabilitation support
b. By allowing patients to avoid working altogether
c. By creating an environment that supports the patient's functional abilities and needs
d. By encouraging patients to hide their disabilities from their employer

Answer: c. By creating an environment that supports the patient's functional abilities and needs
Explanation: Workplace accommodations can support patients in successfully reintegrating into their community by creating an environment that supports their functional abilities and needs. These accommodations can include modifications to the work environment, schedule adjustments, and assistive technology, all of which can promote successful employment and community reintegration.

271. Which of the following is an essential component of successful job placement in vocational rehabilitation?
a. Ignoring the patient's interests and goals
b. Focusing on the patient's deficits rather than their strengths
c. Matching the patient with job opportunities that align with their abilities and interests
d. Encouraging patients to accept the first job offer they receive, regardless of fit

Answer: c. Matching the patient with job opportunities that align with their abilities and interests
Explanation: An essential component of successful job placement in vocational rehabilitation is matching the patient with job opportunities that align with their abilities and interests. By finding suitable employment opportunities, rehabilitation professionals can promote long-term job satisfaction and success in community reintegration.

272. How do employment support services assist patients in maintaining their employment during community reintegration?
a. By providing ongoing support, such as job coaching and follow-up services
b. By discouraging patients from seeking additional training or education
c. By ensuring patients never encounter any challenges in the workplace
d. By removing any opportunities for growth or advancement in their job

Answer: a. By providing ongoing support, such as job coaching and follow-up services
Explanation: Employment support services assist patients in maintaining their employment during community reintegration by providing ongoing support, such as job coaching and follow-up services. These supports can help patients navigate challenges in the workplace, develop new skills, and maintain their employment as they continue their reintegration journey.

273. How do accessible housing and home modifications contribute to the success of community reintegration?
a. They encourage patients to become overly dependent on modifications
b. They create safe and supportive living environments that promote independence
c. They focus solely on aesthetics rather than functionality
d. They reduce the need for social interaction and community support

Answer: b. They create safe and supportive living environments that promote independence
Explanation: Accessible housing and home modifications contribute to the success of community reintegration by creating safe and supportive living environments that promote independence. These modifications address the specific needs of patients, enabling them to live more independently and participate in their communities.

274. Which of the following is an example of a home modification to improve accessibility?
a. Installing a chandelier in the living room
b. Adding a ramp to the front entrance
c. Painting the walls a bright color
d. Installing a home theater system

Answer: b. Adding a ramp to the front entrance
Explanation: Adding a ramp to the front entrance is an example of a home modification to improve accessibility. This modification allows individuals with mobility limitations to more easily enter and exit their homes, promoting greater independence and community participation.

275. What is a primary consideration when assessing the need for home modifications in the context of community reintegration?
a. The cost of the modifications
b. The patient's unique functional abilities and needs
c. The resale value of the home
d. The opinions of neighbors and friends

Answer: b. The patient's unique functional abilities and needs
Explanation: When assessing the need for home modifications in the context of community reintegration, the primary consideration should be the patient's unique functional abilities and needs. This focus ensures that modifications are tailored to support the patient's specific requirements and promote successful reintegration.

276. Which of the following professionals can be involved in assessing and recommending home modifications for patients?
a. Occupational therapists
b. Landscape architects
c. Fashion designers
d. Marketing professionals

Answer: a. Occupational therapists
Explanation: Occupational therapists are trained professionals who can be involved in assessing and recommending home modifications for patients. They have expertise in understanding the relationship between the person, environment, and occupation, which helps them make recommendations that enhance patients' independence and quality of life.

277. Why is it important to involve the patient and their family in the process of planning and implementing home modifications?
a. To minimize the need for professional input
b. To ensure that the modifications meet the patient's specific needs and preferences
c. To make the process more time-consuming and complex
d. To place the responsibility for the modifications solely on the patient and their family

Answer: b. To ensure that the modifications meet the patient's specific needs and preferences
Explanation: It is important to involve the patient and their family in the process of planning and implementing home modifications to ensure that the modifications meet the patient's specific needs and preferences. Involving the patient and their family helps create a supportive and functional environment that promotes successful community reintegration.

278. Which of the following community resources can help patients and their families navigate the healthcare system during the reintegration process?
a. Art classes
b. Case management services
c. Sports leagues
d. Cooking workshops

Answer: b. Case management services
Explanation: Case management services are community resources that help patients and their families navigate the healthcare system during the reintegration process. Case managers can coordinate care, connect patients with necessary resources, and provide ongoing support and advocacy.

279. Why is it important for rehabilitation nurses to be knowledgeable about available community resources and support services?
a. To advertise these resources to the general public
b. To facilitate patients' successful reintegration into the community
c. To provide entertainment options for patients and families
d. To create new community resources and services themselves

Answer: b. To facilitate patients' successful reintegration into the community
Explanation: Rehabilitation nurses should be knowledgeable about available community resources and support services to facilitate patients' successful reintegration into the community. By connecting patients and families with appropriate resources and services, nurses can help address various physical, emotional, and social needs during the reintegration process.

280. How can support groups benefit patients and their families during the community reintegration process?
a. By providing a venue for competitive activities
b. By offering a platform to share experiences, coping strategies, and emotional support
c. By enabling patients to avoid engaging with their healthcare team
d. By focusing solely on the medical aspects of rehabilitation

Answer: b. By offering a platform to share experiences, coping strategies, and emotional support
Explanation: Support groups can benefit patients and their families during the community reintegration process by offering a platform to share experiences, coping strategies, and emotional support. These groups can help individuals feel less isolated and better equipped to navigate the challenges associated with reintegration.

281. Recreational programs can play a significant role in community reintegration for patients. What is one potential benefit of such programs?
a. Providing medical advice and diagnoses
b. Enabling patients to avoid social interactions
c. Enhancing physical, cognitive, and social functioning
d. Focusing exclusively on vocational rehabilitation

Answer: c. Enhancing physical, cognitive, and social functioning
Explanation: Recreational programs can play a significant role in community reintegration for patients by enhancing physical, cognitive, and social functioning. These programs offer opportunities for patients to engage in activities that can improve their overall well-being and facilitate successful reintegration.

282. Which of the following is NOT an example of a community resource or support service for patients during the reintegration process?
a. Physical therapy clinics
b. Financial investment seminars
c. Home healthcare services
d. Disability-specific support groups

Answer: b. Financial investment seminars
Explanation: Financial investment seminars are not specifically geared towards patients during the reintegration process. While they may offer valuable information for some individuals, they are not focused on addressing the unique needs and challenges faced by patients reintegrating into the community after rehabilitation.

283. Which of the following best describes the purpose of caregiver training during the community reintegration process?
a. To reduce the patient's reliance on healthcare professionals
b. To ensure family members can effectively support the patient's needs at home
c. To provide family members with a new career path
d. To relieve healthcare professionals of their responsibilities

Answer: b. To ensure family members can effectively support the patient's needs at home
Explanation: Caregiver training is essential during the community reintegration process to ensure family members can effectively support the patient's needs at home. This training equips caregivers with the knowledge and skills required to assist with various aspects of the patient's care and promote a successful reintegration.

284. How does providing emotional support to family members contribute to the success of the community reintegration process?
a. It ensures that family members avoid addressing their feelings
b. It promotes a sense of unity and shared responsibility for the patient's well-being
c. It allows family members to focus solely on the patient's needs
d. It discourages family members from seeking outside assistance

Answer: b. It promotes a sense of unity and shared responsibility for the patient's well-being
Explanation: Providing emotional support to family members during the community reintegration process promotes a sense of unity and shared responsibility for the patient's well-being. This support can help alleviate stress, foster a more positive home environment, and improve overall family dynamics, all of which contribute to the patient's successful reintegration.

285. Which of the following is an example of respite care for family caregivers during the community reintegration process?
a. A support group for family members
b. A short-term stay in a skilled nursing facility for the patient
c. A one-time financial grant for medical expenses
d. A home modification project

Answer: b. A short-term stay in a skilled nursing facility for the patient
Explanation: Respite care refers to temporary relief for family caregivers. An example of respite care during the community reintegration process is a short-term stay in a skilled nursing facility for the patient. This stay allows family caregivers to take a break and recharge, helping them maintain their own well-being and better support the patient in the long run.

286. Why is it important to educate family members about the patient's condition and care needs during the community reintegration process?
a. To discourage family members from participating in the patient's care
b. To enable family members to make informed decisions and provide appropriate support
c. To shift the responsibility of care from healthcare professionals to family members
d. To ensure that family members become experts in the patient's condition

Answer: b. To enable family members to make informed decisions and provide appropriate support
Explanation: Educating family members about the patient's condition and care needs is important during the community reintegration process to enable them to make informed decisions and provide appropriate support. This education empowers family members to better understand the patient's needs and contribute to a more successful reintegration.

287. What is a key goal of family education and support during the community reintegration process?
a. To minimize the role of healthcare professionals in the patient's care
b. To encourage family members to focus exclusively on the patient's needs
c. To foster a collaborative approach to care that involves the patient, family, and healthcare team
d. To create a sense of competition among family members in providing care

Answer: c. To foster a collaborative approach to care that involves the patient, family, and healthcare team. Explanation: A key goal of family education and support during the community reintegration process is to foster a collaborative approach to care that involves the patient, family, and healthcare team. This collaboration helps ensure that the patient receives well-rounded support, promoting a successful reintegration.

288. Why is ongoing monitoring important during the community reintegration process?
a. To allow healthcare professionals to take a break from the patient's care
b. To ensure that the patient is consistently progressing and adapting to their new environment
c. To eliminate the need for additional healthcare services
d. To reduce the patient's reliance on family members

Answer: b. To ensure that the patient is consistently progressing and adapting to their new environment
Explanation: Ongoing monitoring during the community reintegration process is important to ensure that the patient is consistently progressing and adapting to their new environment. This monitoring helps identify areas where the patient may need additional support, allowing for timely intervention and adjustment of care plans as needed.

289. What is the primary purpose of follow-up visits during community reintegration?
a. To determine if the patient can return to work immediately
b. To assess patient progress and address any emerging challenges
c. To transfer the patient back to an inpatient setting
d. To discontinue rehabilitation services

Answer: b. To assess patient progress and address any emerging challenges
Explanation: The primary purpose of follow-up visits during community reintegration is to assess patient progress and address any emerging challenges. These visits allow healthcare professionals to monitor the patient's well-being, identify any issues, and adjust care plans accordingly to promote a successful reintegration.

290. Which of the following is an essential aspect of ongoing monitoring during community reintegration?
a. Ignoring any setbacks the patient may experience
b. Assessing the effectiveness of the patient's current care plan
c. Relying solely on the patient's self-reporting of their progress
d. Disregarding the need for interdisciplinary collaboration

Answer: b. Assessing the effectiveness of the patient's current care plan
Explanation: An essential aspect of ongoing monitoring during community reintegration is assessing the effectiveness of the patient's current care plan. This assessment helps identify any necessary adjustments, ensuring that the care plan continues to meet the patient's evolving needs and promotes their successful reintegration.

291. How can ongoing monitoring and follow-up contribute to the prevention of complications during community reintegration?
a. By identifying potential issues early and implementing timely interventions
b. By ensuring that the patient receives continuous medical treatment
c. By allowing healthcare professionals to disengage from the patient's care
d. By discouraging the patient from seeking additional support

Answer: a. By identifying potential issues early and implementing timely interventions
Explanation: Ongoing monitoring and follow-up can contribute to the prevention of complications during community reintegration by identifying potential issues early and implementing timely interventions. This proactive approach helps address challenges before they escalate, improving the patient's overall well-being and enhancing the success of their reintegration.

292. Which of the following is a key component of successful ongoing monitoring during community reintegration?
a. Collaboration between the patient, family, and healthcare team
b. Focusing solely on the patient's physical health
c. Disregarding the patient's emotional well-being
d. Limiting the involvement of the patient's support network

Answer: a. Collaboration between the patient, family, and healthcare team
Explanation: A key component of successful ongoing monitoring during community reintegration is collaboration between the patient, family, and healthcare team. This collaborative approach ensures that everyone involved in the patient's care is on the same page, enabling them to work together to address challenges and promote a successful reintegration.

293. Which of the following approaches can help reduce disparities in community reintegration?
a. Implementing a one-size-fits-all approach to care
b. Ignoring the unique needs of underserved populations
c. Providing targeted interventions for underserved populations
d. Focusing only on the physical aspects of reintegration

Answer: c. Providing targeted interventions for underserved populations
Explanation: Providing targeted interventions for underserved populations can help reduce disparities in community reintegration. This approach ensures that individuals from diverse backgrounds and with unique needs receive appropriate care and support, promoting health equity and improving overall reintegration outcomes.

294. How can culturally competent care contribute to promoting health equity during community reintegration?
a. By disregarding the patient's cultural background and preferences
b. By understanding and addressing the patient's unique cultural needs
c. By treating all patients in the same way, regardless of their background
d. By encouraging the patient to conform to mainstream cultural norms

Answer: b. By understanding and addressing the patient's unique cultural needs
Explanation: Culturally competent care contributes to promoting health equity during community reintegration by understanding and addressing the patient's unique cultural needs. This approach ensures that care plans and interventions are tailored to the patient's background, values, and preferences, enhancing the likelihood of a successful reintegration.

295. Which of the following is an essential component of promoting health equity in community reintegration?
a. Disregarding the role of social determinants of health
b. Focusing solely on the individual's personal responsibility
c. Identifying and addressing barriers that hinder access to care and support
d. Limiting access to resources for underserved populations

Answer: c. Identifying and addressing barriers that hinder access to care and support
Explanation: An essential component of promoting health equity in community reintegration is identifying and addressing barriers that hinder access to care and support. This approach ensures that all individuals, regardless of their background or circumstances, can access the resources they need to successfully reintegrate into their communities.

296. How can healthcare providers help reduce disparities in community reintegration outcomes?
a. By providing care that is insensitive to cultural differences
b. By collaborating with community organizations to address social determinants of health
c. By disregarding the need for targeted interventions
d. By focusing only on the most privileged populations

Answer: b. By collaborating with community organizations to address social determinants of health
Explanation: Healthcare providers can help reduce disparities in community reintegration outcomes by collaborating with community organizations to address social determinants of health. This approach allows for the development of targeted interventions and resources that address the unique needs and challenges faced by diverse populations, promoting health equity and successful reintegration.

297. What is an effective strategy for promoting health equity among individuals with disabilities during community reintegration?
a. Implementing policies that further marginalize these individuals
b. Focusing exclusively on medical treatment and ignoring psychosocial factors
c. Providing equal access to resources, regardless of the individual's specific needs
d. Advocating for accessibility and inclusive policies in community settings

Answer: d. Advocating for accessibility and inclusive policies in community settings
Explanation: An effective strategy for promoting health equity among individuals with disabilities during community reintegration is advocating for accessibility and inclusive policies in community settings. This approach ensures that individuals with disabilities have equal opportunities to participate in community life, access resources, and receive the support they need for successful reintegration.

298. Case: Maria, a 42-year-old woman with a recent spinal cord injury, is preparing for community reintegration after a period of inpatient rehabilitation. The interdisciplinary team is working on her reintegration plan. Which of the following factors should the team prioritize to promote a successful reintegration?
a. Maria's level of education and employment history
b. The accessibility of Maria's home and workplace
c. Maria's cultural background and family support system
d. All of the above

Answer: d. All of the above
Explanation: A successful community reintegration plan should consider multiple factors, including the patient's education, employment history, accessibility of their living and working environment, cultural background, and family support system. Addressing all of these factors can help tailor the plan to Maria's unique needs and promote a successful reintegration.

299. Case: Samir is a 35-year-old man with a traumatic brain injury who recently returned home after completing his rehabilitation. His rehabilitation nurse is conducting a follow-up assessment to evaluate his progress. Which of the following areas should be included in the assessment?
a. Physical functioning
b. Emotional well-being
c. Cognitive abilities
d. All of the above

Answer: d. All of the above
Explanation: An ongoing follow-up assessment for community reintegration should evaluate the patient's progress in various areas, including physical functioning, emotional well-being, and cognitive abilities. Identifying any emerging challenges or changes in functioning can help adjust the care plan as needed.

300. Case: Li, a 60-year-old stroke survivor, is preparing for community reintegration. Her rehabilitation nurse has identified that Li's primary language is not English and that she has limited social support in her community. What would be the most appropriate intervention to address this challenge?
a. Ignoring Li's language barrier and providing care in English only
b. Connecting Li with a culturally sensitive support group for stroke survivors
c. Encouraging Li to rely exclusively on her family for support
d. Limiting Li's interactions with her community to minimize her need for social support

Answer: b. Connecting Li with a culturally sensitive support group for stroke survivors
Explanation: Connecting Li with a culturally sensitive support group for stroke survivors can help address her language barrier and limited social support. This intervention allows Li to connect with others who share her cultural background and experiences, providing an opportunity for mutual support and understanding during the reintegration process.

301. Case: In a small rural community, there is a lack of accessible housing for individuals with disabilities. To address this issue and promote successful community reintegration, what strategy could a local rehabilitation nurse advocate for?
a. Lobbying for local policy changes to increase accessible housing options
b. Encouraging individuals with disabilities to relocate to urban areas
c. Promoting a "wait-and-see" approach and hoping that the issue resolves itself
d. Focusing exclusively on medical interventions to improve functioning

Answer: a. Lobbying for local policy changes to increase accessible housing options
Explanation: Advocating for local policy changes to increase accessible housing options is an effective strategy to address the lack of accessible housing in the community. This approach helps to ensure that individuals with disabilities have access to safe and supportive living environments that promote successful community reintegration.

302. Case: Emily is a rehabilitation nurse working with a patient who has recently been discharged from a rehabilitation center. She learns that the patient is struggling to find employment due to the lack of accessible transportation options in the community. What would be the most appropriate action for Emily to take?
a. Inform the patient that finding employment is not a priority
b. Collaborate with local organizations to explore alternative transportation options
c. Disregard the patient's transportation needs and focus on other aspects of reintegration
d. Recommend that the patient move to a different community

Answer: b. Collaborate with local organizations to explore alternative transportation options
Explanation: Addressing the patient's transportation needs is essential for successful community reintegration. Emily should collaborate with local organizations to explore alternative transportation options that can help the patient access employment opportunities, healthcare services, and other community resources. This approach supports the patient's independence and enhances their quality of life during the reintegration process.

303. Case: Carlos, a young adult with a spinal cord injury, is preparing for community reintegration. His rehabilitation team wants to ensure that he has access to recreational activities that suit his interests and abilities. What is an appropriate approach for the team to take?
a. Recommend that Carlos only engage in passive recreational activities
b. Encourage Carlos to join a support group for individuals with spinal cord injuries
c. Assess Carlos's interests and abilities and collaborate with community organizations to identify suitable recreational programs
d. Suggest that Carlos refrain from participating in any recreational activities

Answer: c. Assess Carlos's interests and abilities and collaborate with community organizations to identify suitable recreational programs
Explanation: To promote successful community reintegration, the rehabilitation team should assess Carlos's interests and abilities and collaborate with community organizations to identify suitable recreational programs. This approach ensures that Carlos has access to activities that are enjoyable, engaging, and appropriate for his abilities, which can contribute to his overall well-being and quality of life.

304. Case: A rehabilitation nurse is working with the family of a patient who has recently returned home after a lengthy inpatient rehabilitation stay. The family is experiencing caregiver stress and is unsure about how to manage the patient's ongoing care needs. What would be the most appropriate intervention for the rehabilitation nurse to implement?
a. Disregard the family's concerns and focus on the patient's medical needs
b. Encourage the family to manage the patient's care independently without any support
c. Provide caregiver training, connect the family with respite care services, and offer emotional support
d. Suggest that the patient return to the rehabilitation center for long-term care

Answer: c. Provide caregiver training, connect the family with respite care services, and offer emotional support
Explanation: Addressing the family's concerns and supporting their well-being is essential for successful community reintegration. The rehabilitation nurse should provide caregiver training to help the family develop the skills needed to manage the patient's care, connect them with respite care services to allow for breaks, and offer emotional support to help them cope with the challenges of caregiving.

305. Which of the following strategies can help healthcare professionals address healthcare disparities and promote health equity during community reintegration?
a. Adopting a one-size-fits-all approach to patient care
b. Overlooking cultural differences and focusing solely on medical needs
c. Providing culturally competent care and tailoring interventions to meet the unique needs of each patient
d. Limiting access to support services for underserved populations

Answer: c. Providing culturally competent care and tailoring interventions to meet the unique needs of each patient
Explanation: Providing culturally competent care and tailoring interventions to meet the unique needs of each patient is essential for addressing healthcare disparities and promoting health equity during community reintegration. This approach ensures that healthcare professionals are sensitive to cultural differences and can adapt their services to accommodate diverse patient populations.

306. Targeted interventions for underserved populations during community reintegration should focus on:
a. Reducing access to resources for these populations
b. Ignoring the unique needs and challenges faced by these groups
c. Addressing barriers to care and enhancing access to resources and support services
d. Treating underserved populations in a separate healthcare system

Answer: c. Addressing barriers to care and enhancing access to resources and support services
Explanation: Targeted interventions for underserved populations during community reintegration should focus on addressing barriers to care and enhancing access to resources and support services. This approach ensures that these groups receive the necessary care and support to successfully reintegrate into their communities.

307. Which of the following is an example of culturally competent care in the community reintegration process?
a. Expecting all patients to speak English fluently
b. Providing educational materials only in the healthcare provider's preferred language
c. Collaborating with cultural liaisons and utilizing language services to bridge communication gaps
d. Ignoring patients' cultural and religious beliefs during care planning

Answer: c. Collaborating with cultural liaisons and utilizing language services to bridge communication gaps
Explanation: Culturally competent care in the community reintegration process involves collaborating with cultural liaisons and utilizing language services to bridge communication gaps. This approach ensures that healthcare providers can effectively communicate with patients from diverse backgrounds and offer care that respects their unique cultural and linguistic needs.

308. To promote health equity and reduce disparities in community reintegration, it is crucial to:
a. Ignore the social determinants of health
b. Address the social determinants of health and create targeted interventions for vulnerable populations
c. Only focus on medical care and disregard patients' social needs
d. Treat all patients identically, regardless of their background or unique needs

Answer: b. Address the social determinants of health and create targeted interventions for vulnerable populations
Explanation: Promoting health equity and reducing disparities in community reintegration requires addressing the social determinants of health and creating targeted interventions for vulnerable populations. This approach ensures that all individuals have equal opportunities for successful reintegration and improved quality of life.

309. In order to provide culturally competent care, healthcare providers should:
a. Stereotype patients based on their cultural backgrounds
b. Develop an understanding of the cultural beliefs and practices of the diverse populations they serve
c. Make assumptions about patients' preferences based on their ethnicity or nationality
d. Overlook patients' unique cultural needs during the care planning process

Answer: b. Develop an understanding of the cultural beliefs and practices of the diverse populations they serve
Explanation: Providing culturally competent care requires healthcare providers to develop an understanding of the cultural beliefs and practices of the diverse populations they serve. This knowledge allows providers to adapt their care practices to better meet the needs of patients from various cultural backgrounds, ultimately promoting health equity and reducing disparities.

310. Which of the following conditions may require specialized knowledge or skills in rehabilitation nursing?
a. Common cold
b. Seasonal allergies
c. Traumatic brain injury
d. Sunburn

Answer: c. Traumatic brain injury
Explanation: Traumatic brain injury is a complex condition that may result in various physical, cognitive, and emotional impairments. Rehabilitation nursing plays a critical role in addressing these challenges and promoting recovery for patients with traumatic brain injuries. Nurses should possess specialized knowledge and skills to effectively care for these patients.

311. In which of the following settings is specialized knowledge or skills in rehabilitation nursing particularly important?
a. Primary care clinic
b. Inpatient rehabilitation facility
c. Dentist's office
d. Retail pharmacy

Answer: b. Inpatient rehabilitation facility
Explanation: Inpatient rehabilitation facilities provide intensive rehabilitation services for patients recovering from various conditions and injuries. Nurses working in these settings should possess specialized knowledge and skills in rehabilitation nursing to address patients' unique needs and promote optimal recovery outcomes.

312. When caring for pediatric patients in a rehabilitation setting, nurses should:
a. Provide care that is identical to adult patients
b. Be knowledgeable about the unique needs and developmental considerations of children
c. Ignore the concerns of the child's family members
d. Rely solely on medical interventions without considering psychosocial factors

Answer: b. Be knowledgeable about the unique needs and developmental considerations of children
Explanation: Pediatric patients require specialized care that considers their unique needs and developmental considerations. Nurses caring for children in rehabilitation settings should have an understanding of these factors and adapt their care practices accordingly.

313. A rehabilitation nurse caring for an elderly patient with dementia should prioritize:
a. Focusing solely on the patient's physical needs
b. Treating the patient as if they have no cognitive impairments
c. Developing care strategies that consider the patient's cognitive status and promote a supportive environment
d. Ignoring the patient's emotional needs

Answer: c. Developing care strategies that consider the patient's cognitive status and promote a supportive environment. Explanation: When caring for elderly patients with dementia, rehabilitation nurses should prioritize developing care strategies that consider the patient's cognitive status and promote a supportive environment. This approach allows nurses to address the unique challenges faced by these patients while promoting optimal recovery outcomes.

314. When providing care to a patient with a spinal cord injury, rehabilitation nurses should:
a. Ignore the patient's emotional and psychosocial needs
b. Focus solely on the patient's mobility and functional abilities
c. Utilize specialized knowledge and skills to address the patient's comprehensive needs, including physical, emotional, and psychosocial aspects
d. Assume that the patient will not regain any functional abilities

Answer: c. Utilize specialized knowledge and skills to address the patient's comprehensive needs, including physical, emotional, and psychosocial aspects. Explanation: Rehabilitation nurses caring for patients with spinal cord injuries should utilize specialized knowledge and skills to address the patient's comprehensive needs, including physical, emotional, and psychosocial aspects. This approach ensures that nurses are equipped to provide well-rounded care and support patients' overall well-being during the recovery process.

315. Which of the following is considered a special topic in rehabilitation nursing?
a. Basic wound care
b. Prescribing medications
c. Assistive technology and adaptive devices
d. Hand hygiene

Answer: c. Assistive technology and adaptive devices
Explanation: Assistive technology and adaptive devices are considered special topics in rehabilitation nursing because they play a crucial role in promoting independence, safety, and quality of life for patients with disabilities or functional limitations. Rehabilitation nurses should be knowledgeable about various assistive devices and how to incorporate them into individualized care plans.

316. Why is pain management considered a special topic in rehabilitation nursing?
a. It is not relevant to rehabilitation nursing practice
b. It is a minor aspect of patient care
c. It can significantly impact a patient's ability to participate in rehabilitation interventions
d. It is unrelated to patient outcomes

Answer: c. It can significantly impact a patient's ability to participate in rehabilitation interventions
Explanation: Pain management is considered a special topic in rehabilitation nursing because it can significantly impact a patient's ability to participate in rehabilitation interventions. Effective pain management is essential for promoting patient comfort and enabling active engagement in the recovery process.

317. In the context of rehabilitation nursing, why is the management of complex comorbidities considered a special topic?
a. Comorbidities are rare among rehabilitation patients
b. Comorbidities are not relevant to rehabilitation outcomes
c. Managing comorbidities requires minimal nursing intervention
d. Comorbidities can complicate rehabilitation and require specialized knowledge and skills to manage effectively

Answer: d. Comorbidities can complicate rehabilitation and require specialized knowledge and skills to manage effectively

Explanation: Management of complex comorbidities is a special topic in rehabilitation nursing because these conditions can complicate rehabilitation and require specialized knowledge and skills to manage effectively. Rehabilitation nurses must be equipped to address the unique challenges presented by comorbidities and optimize patient outcomes.

318. Which of the following special topics in rehabilitation nursing focuses on addressing the unique needs of different cultural, racial, and ethnic groups?
a. Pharmacology
b. Wound care
c. Cultural competence in rehabilitation nursing
d. Infection control

Answer: c. Cultural competence in rehabilitation nursing

Explanation: Cultural competence in rehabilitation nursing is a special topic that focuses on addressing the unique needs of different cultural, racial, and ethnic groups. Rehabilitation nurses should be aware of cultural differences and develop the skills necessary to provide culturally sensitive care, fostering trust and collaboration with diverse patient populations.

319. Why is the topic of sexuality and intimacy considered a special topic in rehabilitation nursing?
a. Sexuality and intimacy are not relevant to rehabilitation nursing
b. Addressing sexuality and intimacy requires minimal nursing intervention
c. Sexuality and intimacy are important aspects of quality of life that may be affected by illness or injury
d. Rehabilitation nurses should not discuss sexuality and intimacy with patients

Answer: c. Sexuality and intimacy are important aspects of quality of life that may be affected by illness or injury

Explanation: Sexuality and intimacy are considered special topics in rehabilitation nursing because they are important aspects of quality of life that may be affected by illness or injury. Rehabilitation nurses should be prepared to address these topics with sensitivity and support, providing education and resources to help patients navigate potential challenges in this area.

As you prepare for your upcoming exam, remember that throughout this study guide, we have covered a diverse range of topics within rehabilitation nursing. These topics are essential to providing comprehensive, compassionate, and effective care to patients facing various challenges in their rehabilitation journey. You've gained insights into the rehabilitation nursing process, community reintegration, addressing barriers, assessing readiness, and developing personalized care plans.

Additionally, we delved into the importance of physical and occupational therapy, psychosocial support, vocational rehabilitation, accessible housing, and the utilization of community resources. We also emphasized the significance of family education and support, ongoing monitoring, promoting health equity, reducing disparities, and addressing the unique needs of specific patient populations. This knowledge is crucial to your success as a rehabilitation nurse, and we believe that you are well-equipped to excel in your exam.

As you continue your studies and move closer to your exam date, remember to believe in yourself and your ability to make a difference in the lives of those you serve. Your dedication to mastering these topics demonstrates your commitment to providing the highest quality of care to your patients. By focusing on their dreams, justifying their failures, allaying their fears, confirming their suspicions, and helping them face their challenges, you are making a lasting impact on their lives.

We wish you the best of luck in your upcoming exam and your future as a rehabilitation nurse. Remember, you are part of a community of professionals dedicated to helping individuals regain their independence, restore their quality of life, and overcome obstacles. Keep believing in your dreams and the dreams of your patients, and continue to be the caring, compassionate, and skilled nurse that they need.

Printed in the USA
CPSIA information can be obtained
at www.ICGtesting.com
LVHW011458041123
763047LV00070B/1185

9 781088 212578